5TO

SECOND OPINION

y Myron K. Denney, M.D., F.A.C.S.

this book I will take the mystery out of surgery, describe what
geons are really like, and clarify when you should and should
 have an operation. I will have to talk about unnecessary
gery, incompetent surgeons, and operative failure. But when
m finished, you will have the most complete and honest
:ond opinion' you could ever obtain. And you will have learned
/ to make the final decision about surgery for yourself! If you
 loved one does have surgery, this book will help the opera-
 and the recovery to be a success."

                                          –Dr. Myron K. Denney

SECOND OPINION

SECOND OPINION

by Myron K. Denney, M.D., F.A.C.S.

Publishers • GROSSET & DUNLAP • New York
A FILMWAYS COMPANY

For Leonie

Contents

2115772

Introduction

A few years ago a Russian surgeon, using mirrors and local anesthetic, successfully removed his own appendix. No one knows why he undertook such a bizarre feat. Some have suggested that the man was just an egotistical doctor who believed himself to be the greatest surgeon in the world and reasoned that he should have only the very best for his own operation. Whatever that surgeon's motivations were, his operation remains to this day the pinnacle of do-it-yourself surgery.

Few among us, even skilled surgeons, feel any inclination to repeat such death-defying surgical acrobatics. Yet, if confronted with the advice to have an operation, most of us, suddenly transformed from self-sufficient people into relatively helpless patients, would wish to have more to say about what was going to happen. But, although most people feel free to ask doctors the facts about diabetes, arthritis, or high blood pressure, few feel comfortable discussing the mystical realm of surgery in which opening, repairing, and healing of the human body seem almost miraculous.

Consequently, most patients simply accept their doctors' advice to have operations as "godlike" proclamations and follow orders like lambs being led to slaughter, lying down upon operating tables and willingly allowing themselves to be rendered unconscious and cut open with knives by men and women who are almost complete strangers.

Patients who do strive to learn more about forthcoming surgical procedures ordinarily encounter almost insurmountable obstacles. Bookstores and libraries carry only meager and superficial references, and friends or relatives don't have enough knowledge to be helpful. To make matters worse, surgeons are not known for their ability to communicate well with patients.

To be sure, many surgeons are simply too busy to take time for careful explanations. But even those doctors who try, often find that translating medical terminology into terms understandable to lay persons is an art in itself. Also, under the current threat of legal liability, many doctors answer questions defensively, couching their words in noncommital phrases.

Moreover, many surgeons actually believe that patients do not want to know the facts about surgery. They believe that patients will be frightened if they know that diagnosis and treatment are not 100 percent accurate and that all operations involve sometimes unavoidable complications.

In recent studies, patients were highly enthusiastic about pamphlets prepared to give complete and candid appraisals of the benefits, risks, and complications of operations. In sharp contrast, the great majority of doctors who were asked about using those same booklets in their practices said that their patients did not want such detailed information and might only be frightened, even dissuaded from having necessary therapy.

Trying to obtain information about medical treatment can even be disastrous. Ordinarily, patients in hospitals simply follow the routine, accepting diagnostic tests and therapeutic programs without any fuss. They sign legal documents without reading them and accept doctors' and nurses' instructions without so much as a question. Consequently, those patients who do try to gain information are often looked upon as troublemakers. When patients ask too many questions or take time to read the legal documents they are asked to sign, a pall usually falls upon the activities. Doctors and nurses often view such patients as threatening intruders and potential legal adversaries.

One prominent attorney was virtually thrown out of a reputable New York hospital because he asked too many questions and demanded to have something to say about his treatment. Even though the man was suffering from a rare cancerous tumor, the doctors and nurses refused treatment because they felt the man wanted to have too much to say about his own care. Confrontations over doctors' versus patients' rights occur every day in almost every hospital in the country. Despite the fact that Americans have a constitutional right to be thoroughly informed about their illnesses and proposed therapy and to participate in decisions about their cases, the medical community simply does not respond to or provide for that important aspect of patient care.

With the state of surgery what it is today, it seems that most patients who want to know more about surgical procedures will have to find sources in addition to their surgeons. But perhaps that is as it should be. The delicate trust between patient and doctor just before an operation may well be better left undisturbed by talk of possible dread consequences. Coming from surgeons, information about surgical errors and possible untoward results might sound like confessions of inadequacy. Yet, as more and more people discover that they wish to be more involved in their own health care, the need for information increases.

In this book, I will try to prepare you for the day when you or a member of your family might be advised to have an operation. I will try to take the mystery out of surgery, to discuss in everyday language what surgery really means and entails, to describe what surgeons are like and how they practice, and to clarify the indications and contraindications for operations. In short, I would like to give you a complete and honest "second opinion." To do so, I will have to talk about unnecessary surgery, incompetent surgeons, operative failure, and death rates.

Although thinking about risks of surgery can be alarming, the vague fear of the unknown that so many people experience when they undergo an operation can be overcome. Furthermore, a growing body of evidence, largely neglected by the medical profession, indicates that patients, even children, fare much better both physically and psychologically when they are thoroughly informed about unpleasant or untoward aspects of surgery beforehand.

But even more important—there is information in this book that it is *your legal right* to know. For instance, do you know that judgments by the Supreme Court of the United States and many state courts have ruled that physicians who operate upon patients without informing them beforehand of all substantive alternatives, risks, and complications are liable? Physicians who have been sued under such circumstances have been found guilty of failure in their fiduciary obligations, negligence, and even assault and battery.

In 1905 in Minnesota, a doctor was held liable for battery when he operated upon a patient's left ear after the woman had agreed to treatment on her right ear. After the patient was anesthetized, the doctor had seen that the left ear was more diseased than the right. In 1906 in Illinois, a woman who had agreed only to a specific operation, won her case in court after her surgeon extended the procedure to include the removal of her diseased womb and ovaries.

In each of these cases the operations were considered medically necessary. The surgeons had exercised reasonable judgment about disease, but they had failed to respect the rights of the individuals operated upon. The patients were ruled to have been wrongfully injured because they were not advised beforehand of the possible problems and consequences. Since that time, after hundreds of cases in which patients have been maimed without having been advised of the risks, the doctrine of informed consent has evolved.

Although in practice the law is rarely fulfilled to the letter, doctors are required to tell patients about all substantive alternatives, risks, and complications of proposed operative procedures so that patients can make *informed* decisions and give *informed* consent. If you would like to avoid having yourself or one of your family awaken from an anesthetic to face unexpectedly the loss of an arm or leg, permanent paralysis, inability to have normal digestion, cessation of normal bowel movements, impotency, or sterility, you would do well to become informed about surgery and to find out more about a specific operation when it is recommended.

It's really not so difficult. Take away the scientific jargon, cut through the mystique, and you'll find the principles of surgery relatively easy to understand. To start with, you might be interested to know that surgeons know a lot less about disease than you think. For example, although there are theories and concepts about the causes of acute appendicitis, no one really knows what causes the illness or why it strikes some people and not others. As another example, textbooks contain elaborate charts and statistics about what chemical imbalances might lead to the formation of gallstones, but no one really knows why they form in certain patients' gallbladders.

Surgeons don't know the basic causes of ulcers, tumors, cancer, hemorrhoids, tonsillitis, heart disease, or any other of a host of problems that are treatable surgically. There are many theories—professors in medical schools can recite literature and quote great historical figures, dazzling their audiences with intellectual brilliance. They can categorize diseases as congenital, traumatic, inflammatory, degenerative, or neoplastic, and they can talk about pathogenesis and pathophysiology, the beginnings and processes of disease. But when it gets down to the bottom line, no doctor knows much more about the true, underlying causes of disease than you do.

The remarkable thing about surgeons is our seemingly cavalier willingness to operate so frequently on diseases about which we know so little. There is the story of the man who, noticing a lump on his arm, went to see his internist. After a thorough examination, including X rays and blood tests, the doctor still did not know what the lesion was and referred the patient to a specialist in skin diseases. After another evaluation, including skin tests and allergy studies, the dermatologist admitted to not knowing what the lump was either. Later, the patient happened to meet a surgeon friend on the golf course. After a brief glance at the lump, the surgeon said he didn't know what it was either—but he would be more than happy to remove it.

That story is obviously an exaggeration, but it does illustrate an important point. There is legitimate question as to whether surgery should be called a science. Of course, all medical knowledge derives from basic sciences such as physics, chemistry, anatomy, and physiology. But the application of these sciences to the variables among individual patients and the vagaries of disease is an unsure craft at best.

Sir William Osler (1849-1919), one of the few famous doctors with the humility to admit openly these limitations, reportedly told a graduating class at Johns Hopkins University that one half of what he taught them was incorrect, but that, unfortunately, he was unable to tell them *which* half. Surgery is not a science in the same sense as physics or chemistry—disciplines in which hard data can be measured and cause-and-effect relationships firmly established. The combined knowledge of all the surgeons in the world would constitute only a fraction of the fundamental axioms that would be required to qualify surgery as a true science. In fact, the entire so-called science of surgery might be aptly described as a methodology for treating disease with scalpel and scissors after thoroughly evaluating insufficient data.

Actually, surgery is an art. The practice of surgery depends upon a sound knowledge of disease and careful evaluation of patients, but the actual diagnosis and decisions for treatment rest almost solely upon the judgment exercised by the artisan—the surgeon. Don't think for one minute that we surgeons can base our judgments upon any absolute knowledge such as the laws of gravity or the movement of atoms. Almost all opinions formed by surgeons about diagnosis and treatment are based upon statistics and the theories of probability—exactly the same laws of chance that determine the outcome of the roll of dice at gambling casinos. Fortunately, however, in surgery the odds are in favor of the patient-player—most of the time.

Statistics is defined by the dictionary as, "the science that deals with the collection, classification, analysis, and interpretation of numerical facts or data, and that, by use of mathematical theories of probability, imposes order and regularity on aggregates of more or less disparate elements." A contrasting, if somewhat less exact, definition was made by Disraeli, the nineteenth-century statesman and novelist, who said, "There are three kinds of lies: lies, damned lies, and statistics." The point is that statistics can be very misleading if not used with the utmost care and discretion. In medical investigation and reporting, such discretion is all too often disregarded.

One has only to read almost any issue of current medical and surgical journals to find published articles which are statistically unsound and thus unforgivably biased and misleading. For example, during a twenty-year period in the fifties and sixties, hundreds of articles appeared in medical journals attesting to the efficacy of using anticoagulants (blood thinners) to prevent recurrent heart attacks. Hundreds of thousands of patients were prescribed those medications, many of whom suffered serious side effects and some of whom died as a result of the treatment. Finally, in 1969, physicians with knowledge of statistics carefully analyzed the literature and discovered that not one of those articles contained statistically significant data, and indeed, that there was no evidence to indicate that giving such medication had any effect whatsoever upon recurrent heart attacks. Since then, more scientific data have been inconclusive, so most of the patients who were being treated have been taken off those drugs —but not all. Some doctors still feel that the preponderance of evidence is in favor of using the blood thinners.

The academic puzzle gets even more confusing. Not only are medical data not always accurate and the statistical analysis sometimes faulty, but doctors also frequently disagree regardless of what medical investigations show. Do you realize that surgeons do not agree about such a basic question as which way to make incisions on the abdomen? Some of us argue convincingly that incisions should be made up-and-down, vertically, on the abdomen. Others, just as convincingly, insist that horizontal, or transverse, incisions be made across the abdomen. In fact, a few years ago, in Michigan, professional jealousy and pride were often put on the line between doctors of two institutions fifty miles apart. In one of those universities, the professor advocated only up-and-down incisions; in the other, transverse. Curiously, across the distance of fifty miles, surgery seemed miraculously transformed from a vertical to a horizontal science. The correct answer? No one knows. Perhaps it doesn't make any difference. But we will go on arguing the point at national surgical conventions and in medical journals for years to come.

Surgeons disagree about such basic techniques as when to operate on certain lesions, when to use antibiotics, how to prepare the bowel for surgery, what disinfectant to use, what suture material to employ, whether or not to leave drains in wounds, and many other important techniques that might affect your care. The reason these questions are discussed so much is that no one knows the answers. There is no fundamental science to prove them one way or the other, and the statistical data are too inexact to provide sufficient evidence to convince the proponents of one side or the other.

Frightening? It doesn't have to be. Recognizing the limitations of the art is one of the first requirements to be able to exercise your own judgment about surgery. An awareness of the possible errors in statistics can help you to question the relative strengths and weaknesses of advice you may receive about your own diagnosis and treatment. Sometimes it's simple. For example, there is little doubt that it is reasonable to remove a diseased appendix that is about to rupture, because more people will die of a ruptured appendix than will die from a carefully accomplished appendectomy. But then it gets more complicated. Is it safer to operate upon all people with diagnostic pain and tenderness, not knowing for certain whether they have appendicitis? In this country we think so because statistics seem to indicate that it's safer to remove many normal appendixes than to let one rupture. In other countries, doctors don't agree.

We will talk more about the use of statistics in surgical diagnosis and treatment later in the book. For the time being, the important thing for you to know is that what happens to you in surgery depends upon the laws of probability, because those laws are the most accurate tool we have at the present time. You should know that if a surgeon advises you to have an operation, he should have used statistics to come to his conclusion. First, he should know the probability that the operation will work. After that, he must weigh the possibility of benefits from an operation against the chance of risks and complications, including death. If a surgeon recommends an operation and cannot answer your questions about those probabilities, I would suggest you find another surgeon.

Remember, however, that even at their best statistics deal with "numerical facts or data" to study "aggregates." Thus, although tabulations and analyses can sometimes predict probable events in population or large groups, all the statistical information in the world cannot foretell what will actually happen to you as an individual. In surgical practice, numerical percentages are all too often directly applied to patients without due regard for human differences. Under such circumstances, you would be reduced to just another statistic. Indeed if you are advised to have an operation you may have to insist that your own individual exceptions, preferences and beliefs are included in decisions about your treatment.

Most importantly, after reading this book you should be able to understand or know how to find out the surgical approach to your disease, how your operation should be performed, and what you can reasonably expect as benefits and possible complications. Not only that, you'll be able to judge more accurately whether the treatment you receive is correct and to decide when to contact your attorney if you feel you are a victim of malpractice or if your rights are not being respected. Furthermore, you will be able to come to a personal decision about whether to have surgery and to know what you can do to help prevent problems and speed your own recovery.

Another important value you may receive from this book is the ability to intelligently avoid unnecessary surgery. You will be able to evaluate the indications for operations and discover the alternatives that might help you as much as surgery. The most frequently recommended method for avoiding unnecessary surgery is to obtain a second opinion before agreeing to an operation. The Department of Health, Education, and Welfare is encouraging all Americans to obtain second opinions before any surgery. Almost all of the major health insurance carriers are also encouraging second opinions, and in some cases are requiring such consultations before authorizing insurance benefits for operations.

Both government and private health administrators point out that billions of dollars per year could be saved by second opinions because one survey showed that in over 30 percent of cases the second doctor did not agree to the proposed operation. The American Medical Association and the American College of Surgeons have openly opposed mandatory second opinion programs, stating that doctors always get consultation when necessary anyway, and that because other treatment must be given when surgery is avoided costs for medical care are not reduced.

But for you, as an individual who might have to face surgery, the issue is far more important than dollars. Your very life and limb are at stake. Obtaining a second opinion can help you to avoid unnecessary surgery and the possibility of crippling or debilitating complications—even death. But obtaining an entirely valid second opinion may not be easy. Later, we will point out the many pitfalls of second opinions and show why they can actually be harmful in some cases. However, by providing you with the most complete and honest second opinion you can find, this book can help to put the decision-making process where it properly belongs—with you, the patient—so that when you face the possibility of an operation, the final opinion will be your own.

1
The
Emergence of
Modern Surgery

And the Lord God caused a deep sleep to fall
upon Adam and he slept; and he took one of his
ribs, and closed up the flesh instead thereof.
Genesis 2:21

Adam's surgeon was obviously an expert with an excellent understanding of anatomy and the ability to avoid infection, administer anesthesia, and prevent excessive blood loss. Thousands of years would pass before mere mortals could attempt to imitate the surgical prowess of the Almighty, for it was not until the nineteenth and twentieth centuries A.D. that doctors acquired the knowledge and skill for the development of modern surgery. Those prerequisites were anatomy, antisepsis, anesthesia, and blood transfusion.

The word *surgery* is derived from the Latin *chirurgia*, which itself comes from the Greek, *cheir*—hand—and *ergon*—to work. In the broadest definition, perhaps the first surgery performed by man was massage. We might imagine a prehistoric man, bruised and battered from the hunt, coming back to his cave, and a mate or friend rubbing his sore body to give relief. Applying pressure to stop bleeding, washing dirt from sores, and manipulating dislocations and fractures would have been obvious extensions of such treatment with the hands. Later, tools must have been fashioned to help the healer attend to the sick and injured. Artifacts from neolithic ages include crude surgical instruments which were used to lance abscesses, let blood, perform ritual circumcisions, and to carve scars on warrior's faces to frighten the enemy. Such anthropological evidence has been found in many different parts of the world: India, Africa, China, Japan, the Middle East, Europe, and America.

In Egypt, where medicine flourished under the first great physician, Imhotep, the earliest known recordings of surgical operations (2500 B.C.) were found on the walls of tombs. The hieroglyphs illustrate circumcision and operations about the neck and extremities, and depict the patients as being in great pain. The earliest known written document, the Edwin Smith Papyrus (1600 B.C.), contains over forty-eight descriptions of surgical treatment of injuries and wounds.

During the classic Greek period, Hippocrates (460–370 B.C.) taught medicine on the Island of Cos. His main contributions were diagnostic skills and some pharmacology and psychotherapy, but, lacking techical progress, surgery remained rudimentary.

At about the time of Christ, a Roman nobleman named Aurelius Celsus wrote voluminously about surgical treatment. Since the Romans were more warlike than the Greeks, their techniques for wound repair and treatment of injuries became highly developed, and a wide variety of surgical instruments were invented. The Romans went on successfully to attempt cesarean section and operations to treat hernias and cataracts.

The doctor who would have the most profound effect upon medical and surgical practice throughout the Middle Ages was Galen (131–201 A.D.). The Greek-born physician studied at the Aesculapean at Pergama, in what is modern-day Turkey, then traveled to Rome where he became the most prominent doctor of his time. Galen was a strong-minded, hard-working man who wrote of many miraculous cures but never carefully investigated unresolved questions. For instance, he wrote nine treatises on anatomy, but his work was marred with inaccuracies because it was not substantiated by human dissection. His influence was so powerful, however, that he became the ultimate authority on medicine in the Western world until the Renaissance.

During the Middle Ages, surgery and medicine divided into two distinct schools. For many years, Arabian doctors had taught that it was unholy and unclean for physicians to touch another human body. In Medieval days, that belief became so prominent throughout Western civilization that surgeons and their patients were not even allowed inside hospitals or clinics where medical doctors practiced. Consequently, the art of surgery was relegated to an inferior role and was practiced only by barbers, bathkeepers, and nonprofessional war surgeons.

It was not until hundreds of years later, during and after the Renaissance, that modern surgery began to develop as doctors gradually acquired knowledge about anatomy, anesthesia, antisepsis, and blood transfusion.

The Three A's

Human anatomy first became a science in the sixteenth century when Andreas Vesalius of Bologna developed the art of dissection of cadavers and provided us with the first accurate descriptions of the structure of the tissues and organs of the body His book, *De Fabbrica Humani Corporis* Architecture of the Human Body, influenced Michelangelo and has served as a source for painters and sculptors through the years. Vesalius's work was obviously indispensable to the development of surgery. At last, surgeons were able to proceed with a clear knowledge of anatomy, confidently planning ahead and methodically performing operations. Indeed, in the past hundred years, detailed study of surgical anatomy had made the inner ear, the ventricles of the brain, the chambers of the heart, even the most hidden recesses of the human body safely accessible to the hand of the surgeon.

Antisepsis to prevent infections in wounds or operative incisions developed over hundreds of years. Progress was slow because the agents of infection were microscopic, and until modern times that which could not be explained was often considered the evil workings of the devil. Indeed, a physician who suggested that infection was caused by unseen organisms might have been found guilty of witchcraft. Nevertheless, even before Louis Pasteur demonstrated that germs caused putrefaction, certain keen observers noticed that cleanliness and proper dressing of wounds could prevent infections.

Ambroise Paré was a sixteenth-century war surgeon, not a recognized physician. His original contributions to the advancement of surgery grew from his writings about the importance of antisepsis in the care of war wounds. He recognized insects as possible carriers of infection, and was the first physician to emphasize cleansing and dressing of wounds.

In the eighteenth century, John Hunter, a professor of surgery at the University of Glasgow, became interested in the teachings of Paré, and fostered the techniques of antisepsis in surgery. Thus, Doctor Hunter brought the principles of wound care from the battlefield into the university hospital, where they could be studied more carefully and taught to future doctors. In doing so, he returned surgery to a position of respectability and prestige, bringing it back into formal medical practice from which it had been separated since Medieval days.

In the nineteenth century, Lord Lister, a contemporary of Pasteur, became convinced that germs were the cause of infections in surgical wounds and originated the use of chemical antiseptic solutions such as carbolic acid. Though ridiculed by the doctors of his day, Lister recorded his great advances in his book *On the Antiseptic Principle in the Practice of Surgery*. During travels to Europe the first great American surgeon, Doctor William Halsted, learned of Lister's work and brought the principles back to this country. He developed newer antiseptic solutions and introduced the use of surgical rubber gloves. Always a perfectionist, Doctor Halsted went on to advocate optimal healing of wounds by careful control of bleeding, gentle handling of living tissues, and antisepsis.

By the middle of the nineteenth century, anesthesia had become the most immediate requisite for the advancement of surgery. The knowledge of anatomy and antisepsis greatly improved operative techniques and the care of wounds, but without anesthesia surgeons had to work fast, often upon writhing patients. Prior to the development of anesthesia, one surgeon actually set the all-time speed record, amputating a patient's leg in just thirty-three seconds. The feat is even more remarkable when you consider that during the same operation the surgeon also amputated two of his assistant's fingers. In those days careful dissections were impossible and prolonged operations were out of the question. Since antiquity, soporifics —sleep-inducing drugs such as opium, cannabis, hemlock, and alcohol—had been used for the relief of pain, but they were not satisfactory for major surgery because effective anesthesia required lethal doses. Hypnosis, which had been popularized by Mesmer in the eighteenth century, had proved effective for many patients, but was not accepted by the medical profession because it had always been associated with sensationalism, mysticism, and charlatanry.

In 1846 at the Massachusetts General Hospital, William Morton, a dentist, demonstrated ether anesthesia. The discovery revolutionized the art of surgery by making possible hysterectomy, appendectomy, gallbladder removal, cancer surgery, and all the major operations which are commonplace today. But anesthesia was not without problems. In fact, another dentist, Morton's partner, remorsefully committed suicide after a patient of his died during anesthesia.

After another tragic death, Harvey Cushing, a student of Halsted, initiated careful monitoring and recording of patients' reactions during anesthesia. Together, Halsted and Cushing experimented with combinations of belladonna, narcotics, nitrous oxide, and the cocaine derivatives. Since then, the development of newer and safer anesthetic agents and techniques has made even more complex and extensive surgery possible.

Blood Needed!

Blood transfusion was soon envisioned as the remaining advance necessary for the development of surgery. As extensive operations became more frequent, the number of patients who suffered from excessive blood loss grew. The desirability of replacing blood had been recognized since antiquity, but attempts to transfuse had been disastrous. Greek physicians learned that animal and human blood were incompatible when patients died after being given sheep's blood. As early as 1665, human blood transfusion was attempted, but serious reactions soon became apparent.

In 1667, blood was successfully transfused into two patients, but a third died of an incompatibility reaction. In 1818, ten patients were transfused, but five of them died. Doctors were confused as to why some patients thrived while others died until the turn of the century, when Carl Landsteiner discovered the A, B, and O blood groups, and the concept of compatible transfusions began. Reactions continued, however, and widespread use of blood transfusion had to await further developments. Finally, in 1940, Doctor Landsteiner discovered the Rh factors. That development, together with the knowledge of the A, B, and O types, made transfusions safe at last.

In those early days, the veins of the donor and patient were simply connected by rubber tubing. The transfusion was continued until either the patient got better or the donor got worse. More recently, special solutions, containers, and refrigeration have been used for convenient processing and storage of blood in our modern blood banks.

And so it was that surgery gradually overcame its major obstacles to become an integral part of present-day medicine. Indeed, if today you or a member of your family needed an operation, you would reap the benefits of centuries of progress that developed surgery into a highly technical art. The knowledge of anatomy would help your surgeon to operate carefully, antisepsis would allow for a forthright approach to your operation without undue fear of infections, anesthetic techniques would relieve your pain, and transfusions could prevent shock from blood loss.

Further technological advances, such as development of plastic and electronics, have made possible surgical techniques that would have been impossible just a few years ago. Open-heart surgery, new techniques to treat victims of injuries, and operations to replace diseased organs are but a few of the recent advances in surgery. Indeed, in view of the dramatic success of surgery in the past few decades, most observers feel it is only a matter of time until even more effective cures for cancer are found, more complex artificial organs are developed, and the riddle of the immune-rejection phenomenon of transplanted tissues is solved.

2

If Anything Can Go Wrong—It Might

"Nothing is so firmly believed as that which is least known."

Michel de Montaigne

As a result of advances in knowledge and improved training of surgeons, complication rates have declined steadily over the years so that today surgery is relatively safe. Currently, more than 99 percent of people undergoing major or minor surgery in the United States will survive. Because of this remarkable safety record, most people go into surgery with naive, optimistic expectations. They do not become informed of the possible lethal complications that might develop—problems they could avoid if they chose alternatives to surgery. For most, their operations are successful and they feel they have benefited from the miracles of modern medicine.

However, surgery is far from perfect, and not all patients benefit or even survive. Mortality rates of up to 10 percent are associated with some cancer and heart operations, for instance, and failure rates of 10 to 25 percent are not uncommon in vascular surgery. Such ordinary operations as gallbladder removal, ulcer operations, hysterectomy, and bowel and bone surgery all have mortality rates in the range of 1 percent—one in every hundred patients will die during or after the operation. Many others will suffer disappointment, even remorse, when their operations fail to achieve the anticipated results or when complications result in prolonged illness or debilitation.

17

The following case history is not pleasant. However, this is offered with a sincere desire to help you gain a realistic outlook of what surgery is all about. Although you may feel reluctant to face the morbid details of surgical complications, you should learn about them before you ever agree to undergo surgery. Indeed, becoming thoroughly informed may turn out to be the most important aspect of your medical care.

A thirty-nine-year-old woman was scheduled for a routine hysterectomy. Because the nurses were busy with an emergency, the patient failed to receive her preoperative medications as ordered. In the operating room, the anesthesiologist corrected the error by giving the medications himself. Partly because of the delay, the anesthesia was not optimal and the patient moved jerkily on the operating table for a brief period during the operation. Unnoticed by the surgeons, the left ureter, the tube from the kidney to the urinary bladder, was inadvertently severed.

The following day, when the patient developed a high fever and her belly began to swell because of urine passing from the cut end of the ureter into the abdominal cavity, she was operated upon again to repair the damage. This time, everything went well until a vein deep in the abdomen near the spine slipped from a clamp and bled profusely. In the recovery room the patient's blood pressure dropped to critical levels until two pints of blood were given to restore her blood volume.

Three days later, she coughed violently and her abdominal wound suddenly burst open, spilling her intestines onto the bedsheet. The stitches had pulled through the tissues weakened by delayed healing. The wound was repaired in the operating room with stainless steel wire. The next day the nurses noted foul-smelling, green-gray pus exuding from the wound. The patient was taken to the operating room once more and a large pelvic abscess was drained.

Despite further treatment, the patient gradually worsened and she developed blood poisoning and septic shock. After seven days in the intensive care unit, receiving massive doses of antibiotics, medication to sustain blood pressure and heart function, assisted artificial respiration, and minute-to-minute electronic monitoring, the patient died, her frail body overwhelmed with infection.

An autopsy showed that the terminal event had been a large blood clot breaking loose from her leg veins and lodging in her lungs.

This tragic story demonstrates how complications can accumulate and errors be compounded until the human body can no longer tolerate the physiological insults. This patient suffered problems before, during, and after her operation. She was assaulted by human error, drug reactions, hemorrhage, technical surgical mistakes, infection, and circulatory collapse. Virtually every organ in her body was assailed by the dread complications of a routine operation.

Fortunately, such cases are not very common. But they do occur with a frequency that demands careful consideration by anyone about to undergo surgery. Cases similar to this one are being treated in almost every intensive care unit in the country right now. The grim complications of surgery are evident all the time in every hospital, and there isn't a busy surgeon alive who does not have to treat such problems frequently.

Considering the complexities of the human body, one can only wonder why complications do not occur more frequently. When a surgeon cuts into a patient he is tampering with an extremely delicate physiological balance called homeostasis, a complex system of intricate bodily functions only partially understood by even the most knowledgeable scientists. A major operation is a direct challenge to homeostasis, disrupting temperature control, changing body water and mineral balance, altering the movement of chemicals in and out of cells, reversing metabolism, interfering with normal blood pressure and heart rate, impairing normal breathing, and upsetting the hormonal control of every vital life function.

Even as the incision is being made, the body begins to react in defense. Thermostats reset themselves, volume and pressure receptors signal the vital organs to conserve blood, nonessential systems turn off to save energy, and the endocrine glands release special proteins for the sustenance of life and initiation of healing. As the skin falls open, the protective envelope of defense penetrated, the viscera are exposed to injury from temperature changes, evaporation, and the invasion of a host of different bacteria. If one or more of the insults to the system is too great, or if the defense mechanisms of the body are weakened, serious complications will ensue. In chapter six, I will describe some specific complications you should know about before you ever decide to undergo surgery.

3

The Making of Many Surgeons

A surgeon must have . . .
The eye of an eagle,
The heart of a lion,
The hand of a woman,
The skill of a fine cabinet maker.

Of all medical practitioners, surgeons are the cowboys who ride tallest in the saddle. We are expected to exercise keen powers of observation and judgment, coolly and objectively deciding about surgical illnesses and their operative management. We should have the courage of our convictions, entering where most men fear to tread, actually cutting open our patients to remove disease from within. Yet, we must have the gentle touch to manipulate delicate living tissues and, indeed, to stay the knife when appropriate. Above all, we are supposed to possess ultimate skill in healing with our hands, the seemingly deistic ability to render asunder and then reconstruct the human body. Surgeons, as the admonishment goes, should be the equal of other doctors—and something more.

The father of American surgery, Doctor William Halsted, practiced at Johns Hopkins Hospital in the late nineteenth and early twentieth centuries. He was a dynamic, egotistical, relentless perfectionist who frightened some but was loved by many. He dedicated himself to surgery, married his long-devoted scrub-nurse and worked long hours. Doctor Halsted may have established the role model that has continued to mold American surgeons to the present day. Since Halsted's time, surgeons have admittedly grown more diverse, those of various personalities pursuing different subspecialities: otorhinolaryngology, ophthalmology, obstetrics and gynecology, orthopedics, pediatric, urology, plastic, thoracic, and cardiovascular surgery. But an energetic drive, an eagerness to accomplish readily demonstrable therapeutic goals, and a derring-do approach to curing remain the outstanding characteristics of all surgeons.

If you or a member of your family ever undergoes major surgery, one of the most critical factors determining the outcome will be your surgeon. His clinical acumen, his judgment, and his ability to take care of all aspects of your treatment may make the difference in whether you live or die. But how can you evaluate a surgeon? Most people simply accept their own doctor's recommendation or settle for a superficial look at the surgeon's credentials. Then, if everything turns out all right, they feel that their indiscriminate faith has been rewarded. But if things begin to go badly—an infection sets in, a second operation becomes necessary, or a series of complications sends the patient downhill—the doubts might begin to emerge. If you would like to avoid looking back in sorrow and doubt, you should evaluate your surgeon beforehand—before it's too late.

Intuitively, you know that some surgeons are better than others, and you have heard about incompetent and unscrupulous surgeons. How can you determine whether your surgeon is as competent and as ethical as you would wish him to be? Certainly, you cannot hope to judge critically the capabilities of surgeons. However, some knowledge about how surgeons train, what qualifications they need, and how they offer their services to the public can help you to understand what constitutes good surgical practice. More importantly, an intimate glimpse into the surgeon's motivations, aspirations, and frustrations may help you to understand them better and to decide what is best for you and your family when an operation is recommended.

Training Is Tough

How do surgeons get to be the way they are? Obviously, individuals are not born with the ability to perform surgery. Indeed, most people are naturally timid about open wounds and are apt to become queasy or even faint at the sight of blood or visceral organs. Cutting open another human being with a knife is a highly unnatural act, and attending to the vital needs of critically ill patients can be an overwhelming responsibility. Small wonder that the ability to practice the art of surgery is gained only after twelve to sixteen years of education and training in one of the most grueling programs of personal development in existence.

Those eager high-school graduates who dream of becoming doctors and who enter the premedical curricula of our colleges each year are idealistic young men and women. They come from different family backgrounds and are inspired in various ways; some by their parents, others by priests or ministers or their own family doctors, still others by dramatic portrayals of doctors in books and theater. Almost without exception they are altruistic, dedicated young people who are willing to face four years of college, four years of medical school, a year of internship, and from three to five years of specialty training to pursue their noble calling—healing and caring for the sick and injured.

But premedical education is not successfully accomplished by altruism or benevolence. Rather, it requires hard work and competition—lots of competition. Only one of every seven candidates who begin the premedical curriculum in college will eventually be accepted by a medical school. Many of them will drop out voluntarily to take up less competitive careers. Those who survive will complete a rigorous program of biology, chemistry, physics, and mathematics in addition to general courses in English, foreign languages, and social studies. And they all know that they will have to attain high grades if they are to have even a chance of being accepted into medical school. The four-year program is climaxed by a nationwide examination called the Medical College Admissions Test, which in itself may determine whether or not a student will be accepted into medical school. Indeed, so fierce is the competition in the arena of premedical education that only those who exhibit intense, if not obsessive, dedication to their studies can even hope to achieve their goals.

Of those students who successfully complete the premed program, only one in four will be accepted by a medical school. Deans lament the fact that their choices are so difficult and that each year they turn away many qualified applicants. Some medical school admission committees have even made efforts to establish broader selection criteria to include participation in outside activities such as athletics, research projects, or volunteer programs such as the Peace Corps or VISTA. Other schools try to consider minority and geographic needs in their selection of medical students.

As in other highly competitive human endeavors, a darker side is sometimes revealed. Disappointed applicants have sued medical schools for reverse discrimination. Charges have been made of bribery, influential middlemen, and payola, and faculty members have been found guilty of favoritism, cronyism, and nepotism. The overall efforts to select students who will make the best doctors and be responsive to the needs of society have not been uniformly successful.

A survey of one medical school freshman class revealed that 38 percent of the students had serious mental illnesses, including manic-depression, schizophrenia, inadequate personalities, hysteria, paranoia, anxiety neuroses, and alcoholism. Over 70 percent of the students were classified as immature and uncomfortable with their own feelings. Regardless of all other considerations, one cannot help but wonder why a medical school admissions committee composed of intelligent people couldn't assemble a more promising group of potential doctors. Unfortunately, our pedantic, academic faculties continue to select in their own images, and the candidates who are chosen to enter medical school, the future doctors of America, are simply those students who have proved themselves adept at getting the highest grades in their classroom studies.

Making It at Med School

Once accepted into medical school, the students may feel that the trial is over and they can begin to take care of patients and assume the role of physician to which they aspire. But they soon learn that instead of breathing a sigh of relief, they must gird themselves for even more competition. During the first two years of medical school, another 10 percent will fail or drop out. But the competition is not just to stay in school. The students must work hard for their academic standing in their classes. They all know that their grades not only affect the prestige they hold while in school but will also determine which internships and residency programs they might be eligible for after graduation. Indeed, they all know that the letter from their dean stating their academic standing in their classes will, in fact, profoundly affect the whole of their professional lives.

Some medical educators have advocated a "pass-fail" system of grading, reasoning that medical students have already been selected as the finest the colleges have to offer, that further competition while in medical school does nothing toward creating the characteristics desirable in doctors, and that any further selection is superfluous, measuring the ability of faculties to make their examinations difficult rather than any meaningful difference among students. But such noncompetitive concepts have not become popular with medical school professors, and even those few schools which have adopted the system still retain a third category, *honors*. In effect, students are still categorized as academic achievers versus academic nonachievers. The competition goes on.

The freshmen medical students may also be disappointed to learn that it will be some time before they will see any patients. First, they must spend another two years studying basic sciences, anatomy, biological chemistry, physiology, genetics, pharmacology, and pathology. Their teachers for those years will not be physicians, but professors of science, intellectual men and women devoted to their own particular areas of knowledge and research, some of whom may even be Nobel Prize recipients. The students themselves may begin to wonder when they will begin to fulfill their long-awaited dream of taking care of patients. But they are getting closer all the time. Not only are they learning about disease, but they are beginning to feel like professionals and to understand what it might be like to spend their lives in the practice of medicine.

One essential aspect of professional development is learning to cope with the unpleasant aspects of disease, those visceral realities which may be disconcerting and even frightening. The lessons begin on the first day of medical school when the students of the freshman class walk into the anatomy laboratory. Upon viewing the cadavers lying on rows of dissection tables, some students faint or rush from the room. Almost all of them feel a strong emotional abhorrence to the sudden encounter with death. Most will adjust.

As they take up knives to dissect meticulously the muscles, nerves, and arteries of the cadavers, the students will learn to isolate their feelings, to replace their emotional responses with an intellectual interest, to become involved and absorbed in the scientific exercise rather than succumb to the natural revulsion to viewing and touching dead human bodies. It is a psychological adjustment which will be reinforced many times during medical education and training, and one which will be especially important to those who will eventually become surgeons.

During the third and fourth years of medical school, the students will begin to see patients and to apply their knowledge of diseases to clinical situations. Approximately half their time will be spent on medical wards, studying patients with such problems as heart disease, high blood pressure, arthritis, skin diseases, and neurological problems. The other half will observe operations and learn about the indications, results, and complications of surgery. In the university hospitals where they work, the student doctors will have a chance to observe rare and unusual diseases, many of which they may never see again in their entire careers. During these clinical years, the students are taught by doctors who, instead of practicing medicine, have chosen the ivory-tower university atmosphere, men and women who are experts in certain special areas and who have ongoing research programs.

Isolation—The Doctor's Defense Mechanism

As their training progresses, the students will continue to learn more about their own emotional reactions to disease. For the first time, they will observe and examine patients with debilitating and deforming illnesses. They will see hemorrhage, come in contact with watery diarrhea, and smell the stench of infected abscesses, gangrene, and cancer. In the same way they adjusted to the cadavers in the anatomy laboratory, the students will learn to focus upon the intellectual study of ailments and to isolate the emotional impact of repulsive products of disease. This psychological defense mechanism, called *isolation*, is an essential emotional adjustment for those who must examine and treat disease rather than turn away in disgust.

Finally comes graduation day. At the commencement exercises proud parents watch their offspring receive doctor of medicine degrees, and the students glow with pride as they become physicians. Speeches are made comparing the young doctors to Hippocrates and Galen and extolling the virtues of those who practice the noble art of medicine. A lot is said about caring for patients, about how the young doctors must learn to couple their scientific knowledge with compassion and empathy for their fellow man. Unfortunately, for many, if not most, such admonishments are already too late.

During eight years of premedical and medical education, the students' outlook and orientation toward medicine as a profession have been molded by those from whom they have learned. All too often, benevolent, unselfish ideals have been lost in the competitive drive of scientific, academic achievement. It is as though the isolation of feelings, so necessary for functioning in the anatomy laboratory or on the hospital wards, also becomes manifest in the delicate facets of human relationships. Indeed, the major failing of modern medical education is the isolation of patients as human beings, the emphasis upon diseases instead of upon people.

Upon closer scrutiny, it is no wonder that patients are lost in the scientific milieu of university hospital. The entire approach to medical treatment has become highly technological. Medical students must learn about new physiological tests like blood gas measurements, advances in electronic and atomic diagnostic techniques, and whole areas of innovative therapeutics such as transplantation of tissues; all areas of study which did not even exist ten or fifteen years ago. The sheer magnitude of medical knowledge has become so vast that faculties have difficulty getting all the necessary studies crammed into the curricula. The students themselves are overwhelmed with study assignments. Add to these demands the fact that counseling and interacting with patients on a human level takes time, lots of valuable time. No wonder patients are neglected. So disease-oriented is the training in most university hospitals that patients are frequently referred to simply as "teaching material."

Recognizing these deficiencies, university hospital administrators and deans sometimes sponsor campaigns to encourage the students and faculty to be more aware of patients' emotional needs. One day during my medical school training, the professor of ophthalmology was presenting interesting cases to the students. The professor interrupted his lecture to remind the students that the dean had recently sent out a memorandum to the effect that patients should be treated with dignity and respect. The professor went on to say that even in his own specialty, with particular emphasis upon the eye and its diseases, treatment of the whole patient was paramount. He then turned to his assistant on the stage and said, "All right, now, bring in the next cataract."

In another class, the professor of urology demonstrated a patient who had undergone an operation for removal of his penis because of cancer. During the lecture, the professor reached under the podium and withdrew a jar containing the surgical specimen. Upon seeing his own penis in the specimen bottle, the patient slumped into a faint and had to be carried from the platform. Such examples are extreme, to be sure, but they are true—and clearly illustrative.

And so it is that those of us who hear a certain hollow note in the graduation-day speeches reflect upon the great paradox in American medical education. Although noncompetitiveness, unselfishness, kindness, and compassion are those characteristics most desirable for physicians—and, indeed, are those which motivate youth to seek medical careers—our medical schools are producing individuals with almost the opposite qualities. First, from the fierce competition of premedical education we select those students who are the most aggressive, obsessive, and individualistic. Then, in an even more intensely competitive program, we educate those individuals to be objective, impersonal, achievement-oriented scientists. Considering our system of medical education alone, we should not be surprised that the kind, personal family doctor has all but disappeared from American life.

But there are other, more ominous, results of the competitive, achievement-oriented medical education—the emotional adjustment of the doctors. Although their chosen work is to help others, many physicians need help themselves. During medical school, one quarter to one third of students obtain psychiatric treatment. In some surveys, more than 46 percent of senior medical students were found to be suffering from neurotic handicaps of major significance. In another study, 15 to 25 percent of medical students could be classified as having severe degrees of mental illness, including manic-depression, anxiety neuroses, and chronic alcoholism. The most common cause of death among medical students is suicide. Most of these students pass through medical school without their psychiatric problems being recognized—despite the fact that they are being taught in what are supposedly the world's best medical facilities by the most honored doctors. The problems are carried on into graduate residency training. In one year alone, the obituaries of one major medical journal carried the names of sixteen interns and residents who had committed suicide. The problems go on into medical practice—alcoholism is prevalent among physicians. The drug addiction rate is estimated as thirty to one hundred times greater for physicians as for the general population. More ominously, the suicide rate for doctors is approximately double that of the rest of the population—one average-size graduating medical school class is required each year in the United States just to replace those physicians who have committed suicide.

Specialty Training

Most of the emotional illness will not become manifest until the graduating doctors are in their late forties and fifties when the glow of achievement begins to pall, perhaps even to be replaced by frustration. For now there are more goals to seek—specialty training. Having studied in the ivory towers of academia, 85 percent of graduating medical students will seek even higher achievement by going into specialty training. Many more will return to residency programs after a brief try at general practice or military experience.

Graduating students face a wide variety of specialties from which to choose. A few will never practice medicine at all, but will pursue such diverse careers as teaching, research, writing, music, or business. Some will select radiology, pathology, or public health, disciplines which require minimal patient contact and few clinical demands. Others will pursue careers in the medical specialties—pediatrics, internal medicine, cardiology, rheumatology, endocrinology, and many other subspecialties. In those clinical fields, diagnosis is often the forte, although medical management of chronic illnesses such as diabetes, high blood pressure, heart disease, and arthritis are also a prominent part of practice. Like internists, psychiatrists must also be content with long-term treatment programs and slow, often partial cures.

Of all the graduating doctors, those who wish to achieve dramatic feats of therapeutic prowess on a day-to-day basis decide to become surgeons. Thus, from the already aggressive, competitive individuals selected from premed and brought through medical school, the most individualistic and goal-oriented become surgeons. They are eager to get on with their training and to take up scalpels to eradicate disease. But they soon learn that surgery involves much more than operating-room skills.

First, these doctors must learn to evaluate patients and to recommend appropriate surgical treatment. Then, they must begin to assume the responsibility for postoperative care, including prevention and treatment of a host of possible complications. And it all requires hard work—lots of hard work. Twelve-hour days with every other night on duty is not uncommon. Making hard decisions in the middle of the night without sleep is commonplace. It is as though the word *tired* were not allowed in the surgeon's vocabulary. But, above all, the resident must learn to approach it all without trepidation, to remain objective, and carry out logical solutions to sometimes overwhelming problems.

Sometime during residency training, the young doctors will face for the first time the most profound ramification in all of surgery—the scalpel can also be a sword. A serious complication or even the death of a patient will have been directly or indirectly caused by human errors. From that day onward, the young surgeons will be keenly aware of the harm surgery can do to those who come under the knife, and thenceforth when patients die, they will face nagging question of what might have been done differently. Such responsibility is potentially devastating, and were it not for the grace of human emotional adjustment, few surgeons would be practicing today.

To prevent becoming paralyzed with doubt, the surgeons will vow always to do their best so that they will be able to rationalize, sometimes asking forgiveness of God, when such tragedy strikes. To avoid grief, the surgeons may learn to stay aloof from patients, forming strictly professional relationships, because, deep down, they know they would be unable to tolerate repeated surgical deaths of patients who had been allowed to become friends. Thus, the psychological defense mechanism of *isolation* is brought to bear upon still another facet of surgeons' lives.

All surgery residency programs are designed to provide the experience and training necessary to develop the many skills for total patient care. But programs vary. Some are in university hospitals and are somewhat like extensions of medical student days, with an emphasis on science and research. Others are in private hospitals where the stress is on operating-room skills as taught by private practicing surgeons. Residency programs in public hospitals, city and county general hospitals, and Veterans Administration hospitals provide the greatest opportunity for residents to assume direct responsibility for their patients and to perform operations independently. In many residency programs, prospective surgeons rotate through university, government, and private hospitals. In that way, they receive balanced training, academic learning, expert operating-room supervision, and the opportunity to assume responsibility for patients.

Regardless of where residents train, they should gradually advance year by year until they can confidently practice their own specialities. Upon recommendation by the chief of the department, they are eligible to take the examinations to become board-certified. The tests are designed to insure that all practitioners of various specialties have the necessary qualifications.

Most specialty-board examinations are in two parts. A written examination tests the candidate on his basic knowledge, and an oral examination, in which the candidate is quizzed by a panel of experts, attempts to measure the individual's ability to solve clinical problems and to exercise sound judgment. Once certified, the surgeons are eligible for membership in local, state, and national societies. The certificate means that they have successfully met the standards of the specialty, and it is intended to provide a basis from which other doctors and patients can evaluate surgeons.

The Neglected Curricula

Residency training programs and board-certification examinations are not infallible, however. In fact, many of them leave much to be desired. For one thing, most training programs are hospital-based. The resident surgeons work with patients coming into and leaving the hospital, but elements that affect patient care at home both before and after operations are almost completely neglected. Family and social factors which affect the success or failure of operations are rarely considered when recommending surgery, for instance. Even preparation for operations or the ability of patients to care for themselves afterward are all too often left out of therapeutic programs. Indeed, the hospital-based method of training specialists is one reason why preventive medicine has been neglected by the medical profession and has only recently been popularized by interested persons in holistic medicine, health food programs, and physical exercise methods such as jogging and aerobics.

Another facet of medical practice that is almost completely neglected during surgical residency training is the emotional needs of patients. Just as in medical school, the scientific approach to disease and the rigorous schedules of training lead to the isoloation of patients as human beings. Although the residents are drilled in the principles of surgery, nowhere in the curricula does there appear any evaluation of the ability of the young doctors to act with kindness and compassion toward their patients. Indeed, even the emotional aspects of surgical disease, and the possible alternatives of psychiatirc instead of surgical intervention in psychosomatic illness are hardly considered to be part of total patient care. Ironically, in discussions about the care of patients, such words as *compassion, love,* and *understanding* only provoke embarrassment among surgeons.

Another element that is not adequately taught in surgical residency programs is operating skills. You may be surprised to learn that operating-room technique—the ability to perform intricate surgery—is not included in any formal evaluation or examination of surgeons. Of course, the residents are taught and criticized during operations. But a methodical, extensive evaluation of their skills is never made.

At first, such an obvious omission seems incredible. But there are some explanations. First, many surgical professors are not themselves renowned for operating-room technique. In fact, more than a few famous professors of surgery have been notoriously clumsy at the operating table. The old adage, "If you can—do, if you can't— teach," may have its most appropriate application in surgery. After all, to succeed, professors of surgery must devote themselves to teaching, research, writing, and administrative duties. No wonder that they minimize the importance of technique. Not only that, devising and administering examinations for task performance is an art in itself, only recently being developed by some educational institutes and not yet applied to surgical skills. Consequently, nowhere in all of surgical training are residents systematically scrutinized as to their operative skills.

In fact, no formal evaluation of operating techniques is accomplished throughout the entire lives of surgeons— except when they make blatant mistakes. It is as though an unwritten code dictated that surgeons do not judge one another's work. The concept extends even into medical research and publishing. Almost every imaginable variable has been researched and reported about surgical problems except one—surgeons' skills.

Nowhere in the surgical literature does there appear a study carefully evaluating therapeutic techniques or complication rates according to the abilities of different surgeons. But we

surgeons know that a wide variability exists. We know colleagues who require four hours to do cases that should require
one or two. We observe fellow surgeons who are downright
clumsy at the operating table. But until more reliable methods
are devised and implemented to evaluate surgeons' skills, this
wide variablity will continue to be accepted.

The Business of Surgery

Almost all surgeons agree about one other omission from their
training, one which becomes exceedingly important when entering into private practice where they will have to learn to run a
small business for profit. Cash flow, keeping accounts, personnel problems—all hard, cold facts of business—will occupy
much of the young surgeon's time. He will obtain a city business
permit, lease an office, buy or lease equipment and supplies,
hire a secretary, retain an accountant, pay business taxes and
insurance, learn to withhold employee social security benefits,
and, of course, contract for the services of a bill collector for
delinquent accounts.

As he establishes his practice, the young surgeon will also face
another omnipresent reality of the business world—competition. He will soon learn that there are too many surgeons
around. He may learn that 30 percent of American doctors perform surgery regularly—a number double that of other in-
dustrialized nations—and he may have difficulty getting hospital privileges because the established doctors want to protect
their own financial interests. The young surgeon may find that
his studious methods for competing in college, medical school,
and residency are no longer useful. In the business world, he will
learn new ways to succeed—advertising, marketing, sales, and
customer relations.

Advertising is a problem because it's unethical. Not only
that, it's not prospective patients whom the surgeon must attract—it's the doctors who might refer him cases. Mailing appropriate subdued cards announcing the opening of the new office is one route. However, it also alerts the established surgeons
to the threat of new competition. Another method is giving a

cocktail party to celebrate the new office and furnishings. A prominent listing in the Yellow Pages is imperative. Furthermore, the young doctor should try to get his name mentioned as frequently as possible, showing eagerness to speak up at meetings and in hospital cafeteria and doctors' lounges. One young surgeon actually had his wife call him at the hospital twice every day so that his name would be heard frequently on the overhead paging system.

But advertising is not as effective as other forms of marketing, especially direct personal representation. The young surgeon will soon learn that in the business world, his success will depend upon affability, availability, and ability—in that order. He might methodically go through the Yellow Pages and make a list of doctors in his area who could be potential referring sources. Then, he might make up a schedule, and plan to visit those offices, often taking the doctors to lunch. More often than not, he will discover that the doctors will be polite, but that they have already established their referral patterns.

But the young surgeon must struggle on, trying to impress his medical colleagues. He will clarify that he is available day or night for *anything*. He will emphasize that he would be happy to see bedsores, warts, or gangrene—no case would be too big or too small. Some resident surgeons anticipate this ploy in their training and learn to do some particular technique, such as examining the intestine with a fibroptic instrument or performing operations on arteries and veins for kidney dialysis. They can then use that little gimmick to attract business when they get into practice.

In the doctors' lounges, the young surgeon will learn to discuss automobiles, politics, and religion without offending anyone, and he'll exercise the *sine qua non* of sales—complimenting potential customers on their children and golf scores. The young surgeon's spouse will play an important role in building up the business. For instance, wives' participation in the hospital women's auxiliary, or husbands' involvement in fundraising campaigns will help to build the practice. The family will learn to use every available contact to improve business—church, civic service clubs, social events, and school programs.

As the surgeon's practice grows, marketing, advertising, office management, and sales will become more routine. Indeed, he may diversify his business interests, perhaps even become incorporated, using the cash flow from his practice to invest in stocks, real estate, speculative ventures, and income tax shelters. Professionally, however, he may begin to notice that many of his colleagues have become disillusioned about the practice of medicine. He may discern that the talk in the doctors' lounges has become punctuated with comments about how malpractice and government intervention is ruining the profession. Indeed, he may read surveys which report that more than 65 percent of doctors are seriously thinking about quitting medicine. And he may hear the older doctors say that they just want to make as much money as possible and retire early.

Yes, *the making of many surgeons* is a complex, multifaceted story of development and change. Knowing more about surgeons will help you to evaluate yours when you need one. When you think about surgeons, perhaps you will not only view us as highly educated and skilled professionals, but you will also understand that we have fought through keen competition most of our lives—first in the university for education and training, then in the business world to make a living.

Perhaps you'll also see us as real people, forced at time to accept godlike responsibility, but capable of making mistakes, sometimes torn with ambivalence, and struggling with the emotional demands of our work and our personal lives. Perhaps you will also wonder about us. You may wonder about our feelings —how much we reveal then and how much we isolate them— and how kind we can allow ourselves to be. And aware of our unrelenting scientific pursuit of excellence and the day-to-day financial exigencies of our business practices, you may wonder how many of us will ever find the way to fulfill those precious ideals of compassion and love we so zealously fostered when, as youths, we first dreamed of becoming doctors.

4
Surgery—Who Needs It?

———————◆———————

A free bottle in front of me
Is better than a prefrontal lobotomy

Every year, millions of Americans both need and benefit from surgery. Such triumphs as extensive operations to remove cancer, open-heart surgery to repair diseased valves, blood vessel replacement, and kidney transplantation have offered innumerable patients the chance for cure or relief of their ailments. Even with ordinary day-to-day operations, such as removal of the gallbladder and appendix or repair of hernias and abnormalities of the intestine, millions of patients have been afforded healthier, more productive lives.

By the use of such techniques as hip operations, artificial joint replacements, and nerve transplantation, hundreds of thousands have been rendered free of pain and debilitation, which might otherwise have been incapacitating. Without exaggeration, we can say that surgery has reached a pinnacle in our society never known before in history and still unavailable to most human beings in the world today.

An ever increasing number of Americans will experience a therapeutic or diagnostic operation during their lifetimes. If you ever undergo surgery which results in a longer, happier life, you might very well bless every man and woman who has ever practiced the noble profession of healing with their hands.

But you must have heard about operative failures and unnecessary surgery. If you or a member of your family are ever advised to have an operation, how will you know for certain that the proposed therapy might give you those lifesaving and healing benefits that the art of surgery has to offer? Obviously, to have even a chance for a cure, proposed operations must be definitely indicated in each particular case. Furthermore, the risk of operations must be low enough to justify possible benefits. But do you know the difference between emergency and elective surgery? Do you realize that you have a choice about most operations? How will you be able to evaluate whether the operation you are to undergo is the best treatment for your illness?

To help simplify that seemingly difficult question, let me outline for you the varying indications for operations, from those in which the surgeon's sole and immediate decisions are imperative to those which hinge almost entirely upon the free choice of patients. By learning the range and various types of indications for operations and how to apply those criteria to specific operative procedures, you will be better prepared to assess the efficacy of surgery for yourself or for your family if and when the time comes.

The more you learn the more you may come to appreciate how exceedingly important it is for you to be aware of the indications for surgery so that you will be able to make your own *informed* decisions. Later, we will discuss step-by-step methods for you to evaluate whether you need or want an operation, but first, you should know something about the different kinds of indications for surgery. Thus, you will be able to avoid the errors of those people who presume that indications for operations are absolute, and passively submit to the will of doctors.

The following categories outline the various indications for operations in decreasing degree of urgency.

Immediate Lifesaving Emergencies

Under circumstances in which the patient might die in a matter of minutes, surgeons are responsible to act immediately, performing whatever small or large operations might be necessary to sustain life. For such procedures, surgeons do not need permission from anyone, nor are they likely to be held liable for their actions.

Efforts to restore normal breathing are the most pressing emergency procedures in all of medicine. At normal temperatures, when breathing has stopped for even four minutes, irreparable brain damage results; just a little longer and the patient will surely die. In such situations, artificial respiration is obviously essential, but certain operations might be necessary also. Tracheostomy, an operation on the throat to open the airway through the neck, is not done often because we now use plastic endotracheal tubes that can be inserted down the throat and into the windpipe. But in some cases of crushed jaw or neck, or in conditions such as inflammation of the airway causing obstruction, emergency tracheostomies might save patients' lives. Other breathing problems, such as result from crush injuries of the chest or puncture of the lung, might also require emergency operations on the chest to insert tubes and to reinflate the lungs.

Another circumstance that requires immediate lifesaving measures is the absence of normal heartbeat. Any time the heart stops beating, emergency external cardiac massage must be instituted immediately. Cardiopulmonary resuscitation is performed nowadays by anyone trained in advanced lifesaving techniques. But operations on the heart itself might be required in certain cases. Needles might have to be inserted into the heart chambers, for instance, or a major operation might even be necessary to correct lethal damage following crushing or penetrating injuries. Even laparotomy—opening the abdomen—might become necessary as an immediate lifeasving procedure, such as when a woman who is more than seven months pregnant is pronounced dead following an injury. The operation is an emergency cesarean section to try to save the life of the unborn child.

We cannot enumerate all of the unusual or special situations in which immediate lifesaving emergency operations might become necessary. In the context of your decisions about surgery, though, the important thing to know is that they are procedures of such exigency that you would not have time to consider them beforehand. You would only have time afterward to be thankful if such emergency medical care was ever successfully performed on you.

Severe Emergencies

The next most urgent surgical problem after cessation of breathing and heartbeat is massive hemorrhage. Fortunately, most bleeding can be controlled effectively with simple pressure. Even injuries to major arteries of the neck or arms or legs can be temporarily controlled by pressure. However, when hemorrhage is inside the body there is no way to apply pressure effectively, and such bleeding demands immediate blood replacement and frequently a major operation to control the hemorrhage. Massive injuries from automobile accidents, with crush or fracture of the spleen, liver, or other internal organs, are examples. Bleeding from inside the stomach or bowel is not really internal in the sense that the blood is passed out of the body by vomiting or diarrhea. Nevertheless, such gastrointestinal bleeding cannot be controlled with pressure, and unless the bleeding stops spontaneously, an immediate emergency operation might be required. Other sources of internal bleeding not amenable to simpler measures are hemorrhage from the womb and sudden rupture of diseased arteries or tumors.

Gangrene, or impending gangrene, is another example of a severe emergency. When the circulation to internal organs or to limbs is impaired, gangrene will ensue in a matter of hours. The gangrene may then progress rapidly to shock and death. Surgery is necessary to restore adequate circulation or to remove the gangrenous tissue as soon as possible.

Other specific illness or injuries, such as dire problems in childbirth, certain dislocations and compound fractures, or brain blood clots might also demand nearly immediate operations.

These severe emergencies usually allow time for an explanation by the doctor to the patient or family, but there is little time for delay. If confronted with such a decision, you will have only minutes, certainly less than an hour, to come safely to a decision. Obviously, aside from satisfying yourself that the diagnosis has been made with due caution and that the surgeons are reasonably competent, you will probably have little choice except to agree to the proposed operation; unless, of course, religious, philosophical, or personal beliefs dictate otherwise.

Emergencies

Hemorrhage is only rarely massive and constant as we have described. Usually patients bleed at a slow rate or intermittently and do not need immediate surgery. Their treatment can be temporized, administering blood transfusions and observing to see if the bleeding will stop. An operation may or may not be required later, but there is adequate time for a thorough consideration of all aspects of the case: the patient's overall health, the potential complications, and whether or not the operation is necessary or desirable.

Many forms of inflammation are also examples of this type of problem. Peritonitis or infection in the bowel or chest are examples. Even perforated ulcers of the stomach or duodenum with spillage of gastrointestinal contents into the abdominal cavity can sometimes be successfully treated without operations, utilizing drainage of the stomach, antibiotics, and fluid replacement instead.

Many other illnesses fall into the category of emergency problems that are not immediate or severe and in which some prudent temporizing might prove beneficial. In all of these situations, there is ample time for a thorough evaluation of proposed operations. After insuring that the diagnosis has been made carefully, you should discuss and evaluate the possible alternatives of treatment, then evaluate possible complications of surgery and decide who you might wish to be your surgeon.

Urgencies

Some illnesses that have traditionally been called emergencies might more appropriately be described as urgent. Diseases such as appendicitis, acute gallbladder attacks, kidney stones, bowel obstructions, and urinary obstructions frequently do not really require lifesaving measures or definitive operations immediately or even in a matter of hours. These urgent conditions are often best managed by careful medical treatment and postponement of operations to see how the patients might progress.

For instance, only if the classical signs of acute disease are present and if rupture seems imminent is there need to proceed with appendectomy immediately. In most cases, a delay of operation for eight or twelve hours is harmless and, indeed, may allow time for repeat examinations and blood counts following which the operation may seem unnecessary.

Similarly, gallbladder attacks can usually be treated medically until appropriate X-ray studies can be accomplished. Some surgeons even treat gallbladder inflammations with gastric suction, antibiotics, and fluid replacement until such time as the acute attack has subsided. The patient can then make a careful decision about an operation at a later date under less trying circumstances.

Various types of bowel obstructions can also be managed with watchful waiting, treating the patient with drainage to decompress the bowel, and intravenous fluid replacement. Under that regimen, many bowel obstructions will completely resolve without an operation.

Though kidney stones can cause excruciating pain, there is no need to rush into an operation. Most stones will pass in time and the patient needs only pain medications and bed rest until the discomfort subsides.

Many other illnesses that are called emergencies are just urgent conditions in which there is ample time to think things over carefully, even study them, before coming to a decision about surgery. Although these illnesses can be upsetting and provoke feelings of emergency, there is plenty of time to ask questions about diagnoses and proposed operations, especially regarding alternatives.

It is important to stay cool and think objectively about what needs to be done. Many of these urgent illnesses will resolve themselves in time, and surgery may never be necessary. At least, there is enough time for prudent and careful thought before rushing into an operation.

Cancer Operations

The causes of cancer remain a mystery, though much research is being done. Meanwhile, most malignant tumors are best treated surgically, sometimes in conjunction with X-ray or chemical therapy. However, because there is so much variability in cancer in various locations of the body and of different microscopic types, one cannot speak of cancer as one disease, but rather as a category of many diseases. When talking about cancer, one must refer specifically to exact tumors.

Most malignant tumors of the bowel must be removed; there really is no other approach. Similarly, most cancers of the stomach, uterus, breasts, testicles, kidneys, muscles, bones, and throat require surgical excisions for a chance of cure. However, it's not all that simple. Operations vary greatly in extensiveness, some surgeons perferring more radical approaches than others. For instance, there are four different operations to treat cancer of the breast, some more risky and deforming than others.

Additionally, some cancerous lesions which have traditionally been treated with radical surgery are now managed with more conservative approaches. For example, some well-known surgeons advocate that there is no need to operate on cancer of the thyroid gland, that less dangerous medical treatment can give the same statistical cure rates as surgery.

Certain skin cancers and cancer of the lip also have excellent cure rates with either surgical removal or X-ray treatments. In other less favorable lesions, the cure rate is very low with either surgery or X ray. Under such circumstances, some patients might prefer not to have an operation, but to live their remaining time without the discomfort and side effects of an operation.

So, when dealing with malignant tumors, it is a good idea to think surgically. But it is equally important to know that there are often alternatives that should be considered before undergoing an operation. Furthermore, there is plenty of time to think it over and learn about the specific disease and various forms of therapy. Certainly, no one wishes to delay treatment of cancer for months, but postponing surgery for a week or two to investigate and decide about possible therapy may prove beneficial.

Elective Operations

The great majority of operations fall into this category. They are called elective because they permit a choice both as to when and whether to have them. Patients are not always told just how elective these operations are because surgeons propose the procedures as the accepted mode of therapy for benign diseases that have not responded satisfactorily to other forms of therapy. Yet, these are the operations that provoke the most frequent and vehement disagreements among doctors, and the ones in which the patients should have the *most to say* about what is going to happen.

These are the operations many people mistakenly accept as absolutely necessary when recommended by doctors, but which might be more frequently avoided if patients made *informed* decisions. The surgical treatment of most gallstones, ulcers, uterine problems, urinary difficulties, hemorrhoids, hernias, varicose veins, arteriosclerosis, and disease of bones and joints is elective. Patients should have a clear choice concerning whether or not to have operations for these conditions, and patients and their relatives should familiarize themselves with the correct medical management of these illnesses before agreeing to surgery, accepting it only if and when it seems to be the best treatment.

Diagnostic Operations

Although techniques for the study of disease have risen to unparalleled heights in recent years, in some cases, we still must perform surgery to establish definite diagnoses. In themselves, such diagnostic operations may seem relatively minor — a small operation on an artery to insert a catheter for spcial X-ray studies or to measure heart pressure; the removal of a lump which can then be examined under the microscope to establish a definite diagnosis. Sometimes, more extensive operations are necessary to make diagnoses. Certain lesions of the lungs seen on X ray might be simple benign lesions or they might be cancer. A relatively minor procedure, looking into the bronchial tubes, might be sufficient to establish the diagnosis, but sometimes opening the chest to remove the lesion is required. Rarely, the abdomen might also be opened to determine the source of pain or the nature of a lump or mass within.

Before agreeing to this, you should consider whether a diagnostic operation is really necessary or if there are easier ways to obtain the same information. If not, it may be wise to proceed, but first, find out about potential complications. Fortunately, diagnostic problems of this sort allow time for careful consideration of all aspects before proceeding.

Operations of Convenience

Certain lesions such as warts or fatty tumors under the skin might be slightly bothersome but not threatening to health. When considering surgery for such minor problems, remember that even the smallest operations can result in complications which might lead to deformities, loss of limb, or even death. Patients have actually suffered cardiac arrest following the injection of local anesthetic for removal of a wart. Decisions to undergo even minor operations should never be taken lightly.

Plastic Surgery

Operations for cosmetic and reconstructive purposes can greatly enhance the well-being and ability of individuals during their lifetimes. Patients who have suffered severe burns, for instance, can be helped immeasurably by plastic surgical procedures that improve both appearance and function. However, these operations are not 100 percent effective, and one should learn the statistical success rate and the complications before deciding to have surgery.

Other cosmetic operations, such as face-lifts and breast implants, are performed for purely personal reasons. They are no more important to your health than false eyelashes or padded brassieres. However, patients should carefully weigh the potential harmful effects of plastic surgery against the possible beautifying effects.

Who Needs Surgery?

Sometimes the answer is obvious. Often, the choice between living with the ravages of diseases or accepting possible cure from an operation is very easy to make, and many patients have had their lives prolonged and their suffering allayed because of the techniques of modern surgery.

On the other hand, you certainly want to avoid unnecessary surgery and be sure that any recommended operation is properly indicated in your case. To start with, you can now assess the relative urgency of proposed surgery in terms of the categories we have outlined above. Then, unless your proposed operation is an immediate lifesaving procedure or a severe emergency, you will have time to think it over. You can take time to ask questions about your illness, about the statistical judgments surrounding the diagnosis, and, about the reasons for the proposed operation. Remember, not only is it *your right to ask* these questions, but you will need the answers if you wish to make an *informed* decision about whether surgery is best for you.

5

If in Doubt—Cut It Out

Is this a dagger which I see before me,
The handle toward my hand?
Macbeth

Despite the fact that surgery should never be performed without definite indications, some experts estimate that 20 percent of operations in the United States are unnecessary. The National Center for Health Statistics reports that 66 percent of tonsillectomies, 22 percent of hysterectomies, and 29 percent of prostatectomies performed would not have been recommended by consulting surgeons. A congressional committee estimates that in 1977 over two million unnecessary operations resulted in over ten thousand needless deaths.

Obviously, estimates of unnecessary surgery depend upon one's definition of necessary surgery. Using conservative criteria, some of us think the amount of unnecessary surgery performed in this country is far higher than anyone has suggested, perhaps even greater than 50 percent. Regardless of what criteria are used, undoubtedly millions of unnecessary operations each year result in thousands of needless deaths and immeasurable suffering and debility. How is it possible that in a nation with such a highly developed medical system and such widespread consumer-protection interests the threat of unnecessary surgery looms so perilously? Are surgeons really just unscrupulous businessmen, willing to risk their patients' lives needlessly for profit?

Undoubtedly, a few doctors do willingly exploit patients by recommending, performing, and collecting fees for operations

47

that clearly are not indicated. On the other hand, there is little doubt that most doctors are reasonably honorable men who try to live up to ethical and moral standards and do not intentionally seek personal gain to the detriment of their patients. Yet, even those upright, conscientious surgeons sometimes perform operations that are considered to be unnecessary. In fact, the livelihoods of some seemingly virtuous doctors depend upon surgical practices that if known to the public, might be judged to be highly questionable.

To understand this paradox, we must scrutinize those elements in the system that actually work against the interests of the patient-consumer. We must look again at the practice of surgery as a so-called science and as a profit-making enterprise.

We have already talked about the flaws in the practice of surgery as a science, the vast areas of ignorance, and the unknown cause-and-effect relationships which force us to rely upon statistics and the theories of probability. We have seen how, in the final analysis, the surgeon's judgment determines decisions and conclusions about diagnosis and treatment. One result of such variable standards and subjective decisions is that doctors sometimes disagree. In fact, they often disagree. It has been said that among ten doctors around a conference table any two of them are highly unlikely ever to agree about anything.

The practice of medicine is a highly individualistic matter, each doctor sifting through the overwhelming body of statistics and opinions, listening to conflicting analyses by so-called experts at medical conventions, and then trying to decide for himself what is best for his patients.

A classical example of disagreement and confrontation within the medical profession has been a centuries-old struggle between surgeons who wish to operate upon certain cases and internists who beg their surgical colleagues to stay the knife.

Perhaps the schism that separated the disciplines in medieval days remains with us to some degree even today. For example, for many years most surgeons have been convinced that immediately operating on stomach ulcers is imperative if all patients are to be allowed a chance for cure, including the ones who might have cancer. Internists sharply disagree, stating that such patients should be allowed a chance for medical cure before being subjected to the dangers of surgery. The result is, that if you ever come to have a stomach ulcer, what would happen to you would depend upon whether you were referred to an internist or a surgeon.

Internists and surgeons disagree about operations for gallstones, ulcers, ulcerative colitis, heart disease, and many other illnesses that can be treated either medically or surgically. In fact, internists often find themselves in the role of actually *protecting* patients from surgeons, trying desperately to help them "before a surgeon gets hold of them."

It's even more complicated than that. Not only do surgeons and internists have different philosophies and beliefs about the treatment of disease, surgeons frequently disagree among themselves. After evaluating the statistics and judging where an individual patient fits into the analysis, one surgeon might decide to operate when another might not.

Hysterectomy is a good example of that kind of difference of opinion within the range of indications for operations. Some gynecologists believe that once a woman has passed her childbearing years, her uterus is disposable, no longer useful for any function and only serving as a possible sourse of disease—especially cancer. After weighing the evidence about cancer and other diseases, they conclude that women past childbearing age are better off without their uteruses and perform hysterectomies upon the slightest provocation. Because of this liberal philosophy, over a million hysterectomies are performed annually in the United States.

Other gynecologists vehemently disagree, pointing to the dangers of surgery. They note that during removal of the uterus, other organs such as the bowel, the urinary system, and major arteries and nerves are sometimes injured. More ominously, they also note that unnecessary hysterectomies alone result in over five hundred deaths a year. Those surgeons are concerned about the women who die or are maimed by hysterectomy who might otherwise have lived their entire lives without ever having problems with their uteruses.

Hysterectomy is only one example. Surgeons disagree about the indications for many other operations—tonsillectomy, hemorrhoidectomy, back surgery, bowel resections, breast operations, cesarean section, artificial joint placements, cataract removal, and weight-reduction operations—to name a few. Virtually every surgical subspecialty encompasses operations that can be misused. With such wide disagreement among the doctors themselves, there can be little doubt that many of those operations are unnecessary. Since the indications for the operations are so vague and controversial, hospital surgical supervisory committees and tissue committees cannot control the unnecessary surgery. Consequently, in almost every hospital in every community in the country, unnecessary operations are performed every day.

The problem becomes even more complicated. Even when agreeing about the need to operate, surgeons often disagree about how extensive surgery should be. Do you know, for instance, that there are many choices of operations for duodenal ulcers which vary greatly in their effects upon you? In one operation the cure rate is 98 percent and the mortality rate is 1.5 percent, whereas in another the cure rate is only 85 percent but the death rate is also down, only 0.5 percent. A better-known example is mastectomy—breast removal. Few patients are given the opportunity to choose which of the four acceptable operations they would prefer. Surgeons still insist upon their own choices without elucidating the alternatives so that patients can make *informed* decisions for themselves.

Given the necessary information and the opportunity to make a reasonable choice, most patients would probably choose to delay painful, risky operations until after trying other methods which might possibly prove beneficial. Similarly, if confronted with alternatives, most patients would probably choose the least amount of surgery, especially if it meant a decreased chance of death or complications. Unfortunately, however, most patients never get the chance to choose. They go ahead with the recommended operation without ever knowing the difference. They are never thoroughly advised about the statistics which led to the recommendations. They are not told about the risks and complications. They are not appraised of the alternatives.

Usually, patients are simply told that they need an operation, with little more than a cursory mention of the other important facets of their treatment. Yet, surgeons cannot make decisions about surgery for someone else. More appropriately, the surgeon's role should be that of presenting the facts, of *informing* patients so that they can make their own decisions about whether or not to have operations.

Technical Triumphs

We might remember, however, that surgeons are highly trained people who strongly identify with their role and truly enjoy treating diseases with their hands, and so quite naturally they tend to recommend their skills. After years of scientific education and training, then setting up practices and offering their services to the community, surgeons *believe* in their work. They foster and promote the surgical techniques, some of which are seemingly miraculous operations developed in highly specialized academic centers.

A case in point is coronary-artery bypass surgery. Thousands of thoracic surgeons have now been trained in coronary bypass, an open-heart operation designed to relieve the ravages of arteriosclerotic heart disease. In an attempt to provide precious blood and oxygen to the heart muscle, veins are transplanted from the legs to the chest, one end sewn into the aorta, the main artery of the body, and the other end into the diseased coronary arteries, the vessels which serve the heart itself. The operation is a technical triumph through which surgeons can actually replace the arteries of the heart to try to prevent further chest pain and heart attacks.

Over one hundred thousand coronary bypass operations were performed in the United States last year—and the number is rapidly increasing. Some experts estimate an annual rate of one million in the near future. Sounds good, doesn't it? Well, it may not be so good after all. First, the mortality rate of the procedure has been reported as high as 5.6 percent; one of every eighteen patients died on the operating table or within a few days post-operatively. Second, the operation has not been proved to work. There is no evidence to date that convincingly shows that coronary bypass either prevents recurrent heart attacks or prolongs life. In fact, the only scientifically and statistically valid research to date shows that careful medical management of most heart disease victims give results as good as surgery.

The operation does decrease the frequency of chest pain in a certain percentage of cases, but then so did some more primitive operations, such as internal mammary implantation, which were performed extensively in the fifties and sixties, but which have been abandoned because they are now known to be completely useless; the relief of pain following those operations was apparently psychological. In their zeal to bring their skills to the public, thoracic surgeons continue to perform thousands of coronary bypass operations each week, but one cannot help wondering about the efficacy or the humaneness of offering and promoting expensive, painful, and sometimes lethal operations that have not been proved to be effective.

Another technical triumph, which neither cures disease nor prolongs life, is the surgical treatment of cirrhosis of the liver. These operations entail shunting the blood from the veins to the liver into other large veins of the abdomen. After extensive research, we have learned that such operations can definitely lower the pressure in the veins to the liver, thereby preventing rupture and bleeding. But we have also known for years that the operations do not prolong life; patients simply die in hepatic coma instead of bleeding to death.

By recommending these costly procedures, surgeons make the rather dubious decision that it is preferable for patients to die in coma rather than from hemorrhage. One cannot help but observe that aside from the feelings of urgency to *do something* for patients who are bleeding, these operations are done in university hospitals in the name of research — and in private practice, for money.

The question arises as to whether other highly specialized operations are overutilized. The use of artificial joints to relieve the crippling pain of joint disease is certainly beneficial to many, but is performing such radical operations on eighty-year-old patients really what the procedures are intended for? Sex operations can be beneficial for hermaphrodites or other congenitally sexually deformed patients, but are they really efficacious for people who learned abnormal sexual identity as children and who might more appropriately be directed into intensive psychotherapy? Human heart transplantation, trading one heart for another, cannot hope for more than a 50 percent cure rate. Because of the unanswerable questions about immune-rejection phenomena the actual cure rate is zero. Might not the benevolent instincts of surgeons be more appropriately directed toward research that will eventually help those heart donors instead of actually giving their hearts away to other unfortunates?

History is replete with surgical misadventures, such as mind-altering operations and castration in the name of eugenics. One cannot help but wonder about the deep motivations of surgeons performing such apparently misdirected surgery. Do the patients benefit as much from the surgery as the surgeons do from the satisfaction of having done the operations?

Surgery for Profit

But there is another element in the health care system that encourages surgeons to promote and extend their services. It's called the flow of cash—the practice of surgery as a small business run for profit. In the business world, merchants, automobile mechanics, morticians, salesmen, stockbrokers, manufacturers, lawyers, executives, and public officeholders sometimes succumb to questionable practices for their own gain. In the profit-oriented practice of surgery, how can we expect surgeons to perform optimally? Why should we be surprised if, under the pressures of running a business, some doctors might intentionally or unwittingly advise unnecessary operations that will further their own wealth?

Why should we be surprised if two to five times as many people undergo operations when surgeons practice as entrepreneurs instead of receiving salaries? Why should we be surprised to learn that the frequency of surgery in American communities is primarily determined not by incidence of disease, epidemics, or demographic criteria, but almost solely by the number of surgeons in town?

One cannot help but wonder, for instance, if the fee of nearly three thousand dollars does not have something to do with the extensive promotion of coronary bypass operations—procedures some think should still be considered as experimental. One must wonder also if the promotion of coronary bypass doesn't have something to do with the fact that without it many thoracic and cardiovascular surgeons would be relatively idle since there is not enough other lung and heart disease to support financially the many surgeons trained for that work.

But the same questions arise on the level of everyday bread-and-butter surgery. Obviously, at five hundred to a thousand dollars for each hysterectomy, gynecologists who believe in the disposable theory regarding women's uteruses stand to make a lot more money in their practices than their more conservative colleagues.

Another bread-and-butter operation is hemorrhoidectomy. So prevalent is this operation that some surgeons have been known to say that the world is divided into three kinds of people —those who have had their hemorrhoids operated on, those who are currently undergoing hemorrhoidectomy, and those who will someday need their hemorrhoids operated on.

Do you know the indications for hemorrhoidectomy? Probably not. You may see advertisements on television and in newspapers for preparations which are supposed to shrink swollen hemorrhoidal tissues, but many sufferers know that their hemorrhoids just keep on itching and burning. If, after years of pain and discomfort in and around your anus, you were advised to have an operation to relieve your symptoms, you might agree, accepting the doctor's advice as a medical judgment offering cure. Don't do that. With proper care hemorrhoids do not require surgery.

Patients can take care of their own hemorrhoids by following the principles of care set out in Chapter Fourteen. However, most patients are never told how to take care of their hemorrhoids. Consequently, their symptoms worsen year after year. By the time a surgeon recommends an operation, patients ordinarily jump at the chance for relief, ignorantly allowing themselves to be operated upon unnecessarily. Furthermore, once the patients decide on surgery, there are operations of varying extensiveness which can be done—some as simple as placing a rubber band on the hemorrhoid and others as radical as complete dissection and reconstruction of the lower rectum and anus. The lesser procedures draw a fee of about a hundred dollars; the extensive ones, six or seven hundred.

Hospitals cannot really control the number or extensiveness of hemorrhoidectomies performed by individual surgeons. The surgical supervisory committee would have to interrogate the doctor and his private patients, an intrusion which would not only be unethical but would probably represent an illegal restraint of trade. Consequently, doctors can only raise eyebrows, suspecting that at least some hemorrhoidectomies are unnecessary.

We cannot leave the subject of questionable surgery without mentioning tonsillectomy, the operation that probably holds the all-time record for frequency of unnecessary performances in history. Over one million tonsillectomies are performed annually in the United States — many, if not most of them unnecessary. Appallingly, some experts estimate that only 10 percent of children who undergo tonsillectomy actually benefit from the operation. The indications for tonsillectomy seem relatively straightforward. But doctors do not agree about these indications. Far from it. According to the most conservative doctors, 99 percent of tonsillectomies performed today are unnecessary. The usual reasons for tonsillectomy are: complications of recurrent tonsillitis, such as obstruction of breathing, recurrent ear infections, or mastoiditis; frequent attacks resulting in significant loss of school attendance.

Aside from the fact that the medical profession as a whole has not thoroughly studied alternative modes of therapy, such as prophylactic antibiotics or other preventive precautions in those children who are susceptible, tonsillectomy is recognized as a reasonable curative procedure, and some children have had their hearing spared because of it. Yet, how severe do the complications have to be before recommending tonsillectomy? That varies among different doctors and different parents.

In one hospital the operating room schedule might bear the names of six or eight children for tonsillectomy every day. In a nearby hospital, perhaps one tonsillectomy a week is performed. How can that be? Is one of the neighborhoods full of old people and the other full of children? Is it some quirk of epidemiology thus far unstudied? Probably not. Most likely, it is simply the relative willingness or eagerness of the surgeons to remove tonsils. In one hospital, 98 percent of tonsillectomies were found to have been medically unjustified.

Children have died from the complications of tonsillectomy —severe postoperative bleeding, aspiration of blood into the lungs, drug or anesthetic reactions. In fact, tonsillectomy has been called "the killer operation." Over three hundred children die every year as a result of tonsillectomy; eighteen hundred deaths occurred in one five-year period and no fewer than twenty thousand during this century. Furthermore, almost 16 percent of children undergoing tonsillectomy will suffer physical postoperative complications. What may be just as bad, the harmful effects of a painful, frightening hospitalization upon those young minds is immeasurable. The long-term emotional effects are unknown. Yet, unnecessary tonsillectomies continue to be performed in most hospitals every day.

The fee-for-service practice of surgery encourages conscious (or unconscious) decisions for surgery because it places tremendous pressure upon surgeons to succeed as businessmen. Our livelihoods, the well-being of our families, and our measure of success in a materialistic society are all determined by our ability to make money in the competitive business world of surgery.

The Doctor's Dilemma

Think of the young surgeon just starting out in practice who has difficulty getting cases because he is unknown in the community and has to compete with more established surgeons. He has a strong desire to operate and a pressing need for income. One surgeon tells the story of his first case in private practice. He had borrowed twenty thousand dollars to set up his office and to feed and clothe his family. He had hired a secretary, purchased office equipment, and paid his rent and phone expenses. Finally, after two weeks of introducing himself to potential referring doctors, he received a phone call from an emergency room that the intern had found a patient for him. The young surgeon rushed to the emergency room. After thoroughly evaluating the patient, a fourteen-year-old girl, he decided that she had acute appendicitis and recommended an operation, to which the parents agreed.

The young doctor knew that the diagnosis of appendicitis was often difficult. He knew that despite all tests, blood counts, and X rays, in the final analysis, the diagnosis rested upon his own judgment. He knew, too, that sometimes the diagnosis of appendicitis could be impossible and it was considered perfectly good surgical practice to remove a normal appendix on occasion. Therefore, he knew that the surgical supervisory committee or the tissue committee would not criticize him for removing a normal appendix.

But the young surgeon was an honest man. He reckoned that his judgment might have unconsciously been affected by the fact that he dearly wanted and needed to do an operation, that he was new to the hospital and wanted to show the other doctors that he could operate, that he could go into the operating room and heal with his hands like any of the other surgeons on the staff.

Furthermore, he realized that in the back of his mind was the nagging awareness that for the first time in his life he was deeply in debt without any income whatsoever with which to repay his loans. His wife was getting nervous, knowing that some money would have to start coming in soon. His friends and family were watching to see if he was going to become a successful practitioner. He himself had lain awake a few nights wondering whether in the competitive world of surgical practice he would be able to survive.

And so it was that in the locker room as he changed clothes to go into the operating suite, the young surgeon pondered whether his decision to operate upon that fourteen-year-old girl was made with the professional objectivity he had sworn to uphold. He remembered that during his residency, and later as assistant professor of surgery at the university hospital, when he worked for a salary, his decisions had always been based purely upon the merits of the case. He wondered if, in the competitive business world, he would be able to maintain those high professional and ethical standards.

He wondered, indeed, had his young patient been his own daughter, if he would have so readily recommended major surgery. The young surgeon pulled himself together, reminding himself that he could only do his best. He pushed the doubts out of his mind and went into the operating room to perform the appendectomy upon the young girl.

Think, too, of the established surgeon whose practice may be threatened because a few new young surgeons with fresh ideas have moved into offices nearby. The older man has heavy financial commitments, with an expensive home, a yacht, perhaps a condominium in the mountains or at the seashore. Furthermore, his youngest daughter will be starting college in the fall, making a total of three offspring with university expenses. To make matters worse, the surgeon has just lost a few thousand dollars in his investment in cattle feed, and the stock market has hit a new low. Can we expect that man to be able to make unbiased, unselfish decisions about questionable operations with vague indications that would bring thousands of dollars into his accounts receivable? How many doctors would be able to remain completely objective under such circumstances? Most of them? We hope so. All of them? Certainly not.

Indeed, as we consider the inexactitudes of the so-called science of surgery as they are applied by surgeon-entrepreneur, we cannot help but wonder if the private practice of surgery represents the ultimate conflict of interest. We consider it highly unethical, for instance, for a judge to make decisions from the bench favoring a corporation in which he has a financial interest. We have ousted public officials from office when they have been found to have voted to allocate funds to companies from which they have received kickbacks or in which they hold part ownership. Yet, each and every week, hundreds of thousands of patients are told to have operations and then at the risk of their very lives are placed upon operating tables and cut open with scalpels by surgeons who have personal, selfish, sometimes demanding financial interests that hinge upon important and critical decisions in those cases.

6

If Anything Else Can Go Wrong—It Might

Surgical complications are not easy to talk about because potentially harmful consequences can seem imminent even though they are rare. Consequently, a few patients do not wish to be informed about possible dread results of operations. But in our educated society, most people prefer to gain realistic expectations rather than live with the fear of the unknown.

In recent studies, for instance, women who read booklets about the benefits, risks, and complications of hysterectomy expressed enthusiasm for the information and actually experienced decreased anxiety after their operations as compared to women who were not informed. Thinking about complications before an operation might be disturbing, but apparently most people are happier knowing the facts.

If you could spend a few days on a surgical ward or attend a hospital death-and-complications conference, you would come to know that complications are real and that there is no sense hiding them or pretending they don't exist. On the contrary, before agreeing to any operation you should find out about the risks, then carefully weigh them against possible benefits.

In fact, when you sign the legal consent form for an operation, you are in effect acknowledging that you have already been completely informed of all substantive risks and complications of the proposed procedure. To help you understand the risks of surgery, the following paragraphs will outline the various possible complications—human error, drug reactions, hemorrhage, infection, nonhealing, blood transfusion reactions, psychological sequelae, and circulatory and systemic problems. As we shall see, these complications often occur in combination, one problem leading to others.

Human Error

A fifty-year-old woman was undergoing a breast biopsy to determine whether a lump was benign or malignant— adenocarcinoma. After examining the tissue under the microscope, the pathologist reported through the operating room intercom that the tissue "had no carcinoma." Inside, the waiting surgeon heard that the tissue was "adenocarcinoma" and promptly performed radical surgery, removing the woman's breast.

Meticulous care must be given to every detail in operating rooms. Miscommunications, mixups, miscounting sponges, lost instruments, even explosions can all lead to disastrous consequences. After all, like everyone, orderlies, nurses, anesthesiologists, and surgeons have their bad days. With the complexities of operating room procedures, any breakdown in routine disrupts the teamwork and can lead to serious complications.

There isn't a surgeon in practice who doesn't make technical errors during operations. Sometimes we cut the wrong structure, sometimes we tie the wrong tissue, or commit any number of so-called oopsies. Fictional stories often dramatize such mistakes, but in real life they happen all the time. Almost no operation is complete without some small, inconsequential errors. But when sharp steel instruments are repeatedly brought into contact with delicate, living tissues, some serious technical errors are almost inevitable. Fortunately, mistakes during operations are usually recognized and corrected immediately. When they go unnoticed, however, they can lead to serious consequences.

Drug Reaction

A seven-year-old boy was admitted to the hospital for a routine tonsillectomy. On the morning of his operation, the nurse gave the patient an injection, a drug to relieve anxiety. Fifteen minutes later, the boy broke out in a rash and his throat began to swell so that his respirations came in labored gasps. Heroic measures were required to save the boy's life.

This patient was allergic to the medication. Like most serious drug allergies, the complication struck suddenly and without warning. But patients also suffer from other side reactions to drugs.

In the recovery room following hemorrhoidectomy, a fifty-year-old man became restless, pulling at his bedclothes and trying to climb over the rails of the stretcher. The nurse called the surgeon who ordered additional pain medication and a tranquilizer. Fifteen minutes later, the man died in his bed and resuscitative efforts failed.

In this all-too-common postoperative complication, the patient died as a result of the side effects and misuse of drugs. All pain medications and anesthetic gases depress normal respirations. The doctor in this case failed to recognize that the patient's irritability and restlessness were not because of pain, but were caused by decreased respirations leading to lowered oxygen content in the blood, hypoxia. The additional medication only made the problem worse, lowering the brain's oxygen to critical levels.

Hemorrhage

A fifty-year-old man was undergoing a bronchoscopy, a special diagnostic examination to look into the larynx and bronchial tubes. The surgeon decided to perform a biopsy, to take a small piece of tissue for microscopic examination. As the sharp teeth of the biopsy forceps closed on the tissue, blood suddenly welled up uncontrollably, pouring from the man's mouth. In a matter of minutes, he drowned in his own blood.

Here is a case of massive hemorrhage caused by our old friend human error. The surgeon obviously cut the wrong structure. The "tumor" he biopsied was in reality a large blood vessel leading to the heart. The cause of the hemorrhage was painfully obvious. Indeed, Doctor Halsted once said, "The only weapon with which the unconscious patient can immediately retaliate upon the incompetent surgeon is hemorrhage. If he bleeds to death, it may be presumed that the surgeon is to blame . . . ." In other cases, however, the cause of hemorrhage may not be so obvious.

A forty-five-year-old woman underwent a hysterectomy. She slept well through the night, but in the morning as she was helped to stand by her bedside, a sudden gush of blood poured from her vagina and down her legs. She slumped to the floor as her blood pressure dropped to critical levels.

Hemorrhage is one of the most common and most dreaded of operative complications, sometimes dramatic, but other times slow and insidious, gradually depleting blood volume. In either case, the source of bleeding must be found and controlled as soon as possible, or the patient will surely die. Often, post-operative hemorrhage is caused by human error, but certain operations such as tonsillectomy, hysterectomy, and prostatectomy are fraught with hemorrhage despite all precautions. Abnormal blood clotting tendencies, blood transfusion reactions, certain infections, and vitamin deficiencies can predispose patients to the complication of hemorrhage.

Infection

An elderly man underwent repair of a hernia in his groin. The operation went well and the man was discharged from the hospital on the second postoperative day. At home, however, the patient began to feel weak with intermittent chills and fever. Noting increasing pain, the man looked under his dressings to find copious amounts of gray-yellow pus exuding from the wound as though a huge boil had been lanced.

Despite the great advances in surgical antisepsis since Paré, Hunter, and Lister, 1 to 2 percent of all operative wounds still become infected. Frequently, such infections can be controlled with proper treatment. All too often, however, they spread uncontrollably. Despite all antiseptic techniques and antibiotics, infection is still the number one cause of death on surgical wards.

Other surgical complications such as hemorrhage, human error, and drug misuse predispose patients to infection, as the preceding case histories have shown. In fact, whenever less than ideal conditions exist—lowered patient resistance, contamination of wounds, exposure of patients to virulent bacteria—infection will attack. The bacteria may then spread through the bloodstream attacking the lungs, kidneys, liver, heart, and brain, eventually killing by releasing toxins that destroy bodily function and cause septic shock. Ironically, the most dreaded surgical infections are caused by bacteria that live and grow inside the very hospitals in which operations are performed.

Nonhealing

A sixty-five-year-old man underwent an operation to remove a cancerous lesion from his bowel. Five days afterward, the patient coughed and his wound ruptured, spilling his intestines from the abdominal cavity. The patient was returned to the operating room to have the incision closed again, this time with stainless steel sutures.

The success of all surgery depends upon the ability of the human body to mend itself. Surgeons' efforts at reconstruction would be fruitless without natural healing of the skin, abdominal wall, bones, or various organs. Healing is a very complex process whereby the body is able to rebuild cells or substitute fibrous protein in the form of scars to seal and bind together tissues which have been cut. This physiological repair requires building blocks of protein molecules held together in microscopic networks. But for the protein to undergo such organizations, vitamins and minerals are needed as catalysts and activating agents. Vitamins A, C, K, and E have all been shown to play a role in wound healing. Iron, calcium, zinc, magnesium, and selenium also play important roles.

Local factors are also important for healing. Careful operative technique to bring severed surfaces together firmly and cleanly without interfering with precious blood supply is necessary for optimal healing. Swelling, blood clots, or foreign material at the interface of healing surfaces will block the formation of the protein networks at the cell level.

Most good surgeons pay careful attention to meticulous technique, but those slow, clumsy fellows or those who fail to exercise caution and good judgment obviously become a hindrance rather than a help to healing. However, even good surgeons all too often neglect nutrition and the general good health of patients so necessary for proper healing.

Two and a half percent of all abdominal wounds fail to heal properly—5.4 percent in patients over forty-five years of age. Add to that the number of cases in which internal healing fails, and one discovers an appalling number of surgical complications because of failure to heal. Obviously, continued improvement in operative technique will help reduce the rate of nonhealing. However, a vast reassessment of the importance of nutrition might be the greatest advance toward improving healing in surgical patients.

Complications of Blood Transfusion

As a milestone in the history of surgery, blood transfusion paved the way to bigger and better operations. Nearly ten million units of blood are administered in the United States annually. Without this blood extensive operations would be impossible —the patients would simply bleed to death during surgery. However, like all other modes of treatment, blood transfusions are double-edged swords, offering therapeutic value but not without the risk of serious, sometimes lethal complications. At a conservative estimate of a 2 percent complication rate, over two hundred thousand untoward results of blood transfusion occur each year. Other estimates run as high as 10 percent, and the risk of death from one unit of blood is as great as for some major operations.

Bacterial contamination of blood can cause serious complications. Ordinarily, blood is refrigerated to prevent spoilage just like food at home. But when the blood is improperly handled or allowed to warm, growth of bacteria can occur, and the life-giving transfusion becomes, instead, an instrument of death.

Other diseases can be transmitted by blood transfusion, the

most prevalent of which is serum or infectious hepatitis. As many as 30 percent of blood donors have been shown to harbor hepatitis virus, and the transmission of disease to transfused patients constitutes a serious risk. The symptoms of fever, fatigue, indigestion, and jaundice do not appear until after an incubation period of fifteen days to four months. Although most of these cases will improve, some go on to liver destruction, cirrhosis, and death. Other less serious reactions to transfused blood, such as allergic or unexplained fevers, are usually mild and can be controlled with appropriate treatment.

All too often blood is given unnecessarily, either because of inept surgical techniques resulting in excessive blood loss or because of the eagerness of doctors to "protect" patients by giving "preventive" transfusion. On the contrary, safe surgery demands minimizing blood loss, carefully assessing the fluid needs of patients, and judiciously utilizing transfusions.

Psychological Complications

A seventy-year-old woman underwent an operation for a fractured hip. Although she was an alert, responsive person, two days after her operation she began hallucinating and became hostile and combative. Restraints and tranquilizers were necessary to prevent the woman from harming herself.

Psychological implications are the most neglected aspect of all surgery. Children and adults of all ages experience many different emotional reactions to operations. Almost everyone normally has increased anxiety and apprehension about an illness or an operation. One such reaction is the tendency to regression, in which patients revert to a more dependent, childlike state and look to their doctors and nurses as omnipotent, parental figures.

For some patients the experience becomes too threatening, even overwhelming, and they become depressed and irritable. Others respond more demonstratively, locking themselves in rooms or refusing to talk to anyone. One might think that after the operation anxiety would disappear since the threatening episode has passed. But not necessarily so. A surprisingly high percentage of people continue postoperatively to experience increased anxiety, sometimes even severe psychiatric disturbances.

Elderly people are especially prone to mental problems when forced to leave their familiar surroundings and go into hospitals. They become disoriented, refuse to eat, and may even hallucinate. This state of mental aberration is sometimes called the "ceiling syndrome" because it seems to be triggered by the boredom of staring upward from a hospital bed. When returned to their homes, these patients promptly revert to normal behavior.

All too often, however, emotional disturbances in surgical patients are recognized only after it is too late, after patients commit suicide or become deeply psychotic. Almost every surgical doctor and nurse can recall a case in which the operation was a success—except that a few days afterward the patient jumped out of the window. In the course of operation and recovery, the frequency and severity of psychological reactions are often overlooked.

We surgeons are woefully untrained and inept at diagnosing or even recognizing the sometimes subtle manifestations of psychiatric problems. Indeed, surgeons' training and ability to isolate themselves from emotional expression may actually block their appreciation of psychological disturbances in their patients. Sometimes, however, the symptoms are painfully obvious.

A six-year-old girl underwent tonsillectomy. Prior to the operation she showed increased fears, clinging to her mother and awakening at night in terror. The operation went well without physical complications, but at home afterward the child refused to go to school, began bed-wetting, would not eat, and began to pick at her skin, producing sores on her body. Psychotherapy was required to help the child.

The emotional disturbance experienced by this child following tonsillectomy is not a rare occurrence. Virtually all children who undergo operations experience activation of childhood fears of abandonment, mutilation, and death. In some, the emotional reactions will be severe, impairing normal relationships and function. More ominously, 26 percent of those children with preoperative symptoms will react to their operations as disturbing, disruptive experiences with indelible impact upon later personality development. Studies have shown that nearly 21 percent of all children undergoing operations have serious emotional reactions afterward.

Emotional disturbances caused by surgery can, in turn, produce serious physical consequences. Every surgeon has seen patients who lose their will to live and go on to die despite all medical care. But less severe emotional reactions can also lead to physical complications. Patients who are depressed or anxious and cannot command the motivation required to cough and breathe deeply postoperatively may develop pneumonia, for instance, and patients who do not move about and ambulate may develop blood clots in their legs. The ramifications of psychological implications of surgery are immeasurable, but they may be more important than all other aspects of postoperative care.

Studies have shown that predicting which patients will experience severe emotional disturbances postoperatively is difficult. However, the most neglected, yet one of the most significant principles of the emotional aspects of surgery is that patients who do the best postoperatively are those who have become informed beforehand so that they have realistic expectations.

Circulatory Complications

A fifty-year-old man underwent a hemorrhoidectomy under spinal anesthesia. During the operation, he became agitated and complained of pain. The anesthesiologist gave him more medication to calm the patient. In the recovery room postoperatively the man suddenly collapsed, and despite resuscititive efforts, died. Autopsy revealed a massive heart attack.

This man died as a result of circulatory complications. The combined efforts of anesthesia and surgery superimposed upon his already diseased coronary arteries resulted in a fatal heart attack. The function of every organ in the body depends upon minute-to-minute blood flow bringing oxygen to the tissues.

During operations and afterward, circulation is impaired because of inactivity, drugs, and blood loss. Especially in patients with arteriosclerosis, the impaired circulation may result in oxygen deprivation, then destruction of the affected tissues—heart, kidneys, lungs, brain, or extremities, as the case may be.

Decreased activity and slowed circulation during and after surgery also increases the tendency for clots to form within veins or arteries. Arteries with arteriosclerosis may become completely blocked by blood clots, thereby stopping all flow and resulting in gangrene. Clots can form in veins, too, especially in the lower half of the body. Not infrequently, blood clots inside the veins of the legs produce inflammation and the swelling of phlebitis. If blood clots break off from the vein wall, they can travel through the venous system to the lungs, causing dread pulmonary emboli and resulting in sudden death.

Systemic Complications

Curiously, some complications of surgery occur without any apparent cause or direct relation to a particular operation. For instance, appendicitis and gallbladder attacks occur more frequently in postoperative patients than in the general population. Endocrine glands can become depleted of essential hormones and thyroid attacks or other glandular derangements can occur. More serious consequences such as stomach ulceration and hemorrhage can also occur in response to the stress of operations. These unusual complications are unpredictable, but must be recognized and treated promptly when they occur.

The complications of surgery—human error, drug reactions, infection, hemorrhage, nonhealing, blood transfusion reactions, psychological and circulatory problems—all work against recovery following operations. As we have shown, these complications can worsen and accumulate, eventually killing by attacking vital organs. Some surgical complications are preventable, but other seem to occur despite all precautions. Fortunately, complications are exceptions and not the rule. Millions of operations are performed safely every month. But knowing about possible complications is important for you, not only to give you a realistic outlook toward your operation but to help you know how to prevent problems in your own case. Later we will discuss what you can do to avoid the complications of surgery.

7

To Sleep—Perchance to Awaken

Upon receiving a bill for three hundred dollars from an anesthesiologist, the patient called to complain. "You charged me three hundred dollars just to put me to sleep," she said.
"That's not correct," said the anesthesiologist. "I charged you five dollars for putting you to sleep. I charged two hundred ninety-five dollars for waking you up."

In the United States more than ten thousand people die every year solely as a result of anesthesia. Including all major and minor surgery, one of every sixteen hundred operations results in the death of the patient because of the anesthetic. Considering the intricacies of modern anesthesia for major operations and the risks of giving potent drugs to debilitated patients, the figure is not alarming. But although the number is so low as to escape routine notice by doctors and patients, it is high enough on a national scale to represent a major health threat. A similar death rate for air travel or industry, for instance, would fall far below acceptable safety standards.

Tragically, approximately two thousand of those deaths occur as a result of unnecessary surgery, and many others might be prevented. Like all other aspects of surgery, anesthesia is not without significant risks. Indeed, for themselves and their own families, most doctors and nurses are more concerned about anesthesia than any other aspect of surgery.

During administration of anesthesia, sudden catastrophic complications sometimes occur—cardiac arrest, oxygen deprivation, aspiration of stomach contents into the lungs, critical drops in blood pressure, and uncontrollable fevers. These events can then cause death or crippling and debilitating consequences such as brain damage, spinal cord paralysis, kidney failure, or pneumonia.

Other less dramatic complications can also occur — eye damage, temporary nerve paralysis, lung collapse, inflammation, circulatory problems, depression of respirations, liver damage, and allergic reactions. Literally every normal physiological function for survival is disrupted during anesthesia, and tampering with these delicate living mechanisms is certain to cause some complications. Even more than surgeons, anesthesiologists truly take their patients' lives into their own hands. Your choice of anesthesiologist and method of anesthesia deserves as much consideration as the surgery itself.

Obviously, if you have to face the necessity of a major operation, you must accept the risks of anesthesia or else return to the barbaric, painful surgery of more than a century ago. After all, including major and minor surgery, the odds of surviving an anesthetic are 1599 to 1, a testimony to the quality of the practice of anesthesia. But a surprisingly high percentage of anesthesia results in some complications. Besides, statistics would offer little consolation if you or a member of your family were maimed or died as a result of anesthesia—especially if the risk were unnecessary or the tragic outcome avoidable.

In the nineteenth century, in reaction to the tragic death of a patient, Doctor Harvey Cushing, later to become a famous neurosurgeon, established the anesthetic record that heralded the beginnings of the specialty of anesthesiology. Since then, the risks of anesthesia have decreased dramatically. Today, anesthesiologists are trained in residency programs just as surgeons are. They spend two or three years after internship acquiring a thorough knowledge of physiology and pharmacology in addition to the techniques of administering anesthesia. In most hospitals, nurse anesthetists also play an important role, working under the supervision of anesthesiologists or surgeons and providing the technical skills of administering anesthetics.

Anesthesia means absence of feeling. Ideally, an anesthetic agent would render patients completely free of pain while leaving other feelings intact, but would not interfere with important bodily functions and would not cause untoward side effects. But a perfect anesthetic agent does not exist. Far from it. Every drug used in anesthesia has many harmful, potentially lethal side effects. In fact, the art of anesthesia embodies maximizing the benefits and minimizing the risks by proper selection and by the use of combinations of agents to obtain the most desirable effects. Even then, utmost precaution must be observed to detect and treat problems before they cause harm to patients.

The anesthesiologist's lot is not always a happy one. A great deal of pressure is exerted upon anesthesiologists by surgeons and operating room supervisors to get cases underway and not to waste time. Anesthesiologists sometimes must insist, even demand, the time to exercise the necessary precautions.

In our modern costly operating rooms, anesthesia must be reliable, fast, and effective so as to allow for efficient and economic use of space and personnel. Consequently, time-consuming techniques, even careful counseling, are often not practical. All too often, drugs and gases are used where reassurance and guidance might be more efficacious — and a lot safer. To help patients tolerate surgery safely, anesthesiologists choose from a wide range of scientic techniques and drugs.

Types of Anesthesia

Whatever type of anesthesia you might receive during your own operation, there are many other aspects you should know about — such as the use of muscle relaxants, placing tubes into your airway, and using equipment like artificial respirators. You should discuss these matters with your anesthesiologist or surgeon before your operation.

Good medical care dictates that you be seen and evaluated for anesthesia before your operation. In most hospitals, your anesthesiologist would see you in the afternoon or evening before your operation. Under emergency conditions, the anesthesiologist might see you in the emergency room, or if necessary, in the operating room. During that interview, the doctor should get to know your case, to learn about your medical history, including some things about your family and your allergies or unusual reactions to drugs.

This consultation is very important — it might even save your life. But this visit can also give you an opportunity to find out what is going to happen in your particular case, and to evaluate your anesthesiologist.

Ask what the anethesiologist plans to do.

Ask if you are receiving the safest anesthesia for your case. If not, why.

Ask the anesthesiologist about himself, his training, and his credentials. You have a limited choice because anesthesiologists work in hospital groups, which are virtual monopolies. But you still have some choice, and the final opinion should be your own.

If you do not like the anesthesiologist you see, ask for another. Remember, that doctor is going to take your life into his hands.

The anesthesiologist's preoperative visit should have still another benefit for you. Properly done, it should be a chance for you to have your fears allayed, your anxiety diminished. Studies have shown that cursory visits by anesthesiologists preoperatively can actually increase patients' anxieties, raising more questions than they answer. But more and more evidence is showing that if these consultations are supportive they can have important calming effects.

Whatever operation you might have to undergo, you should find out about your anesthesia.

"Local" anesthesia is the simplest, and perhaps the safest, form of medical pain relief during operations. With it, chemicals of the *caine* derivative are injected into the skin and tissues thereby numbing the small nerves. The absence of feeling thus derived is excellent for small operations such as removal of moles or even fairly extensive plastic surgical procedures. But local anesthetics do have some drawbacks. First, the patients feel pain during insertion of the needles and injection of medications. Also, the drugs produce adequate anesthesia for only up to forty-five minutes, after which repeat injections may be necessary.

More importantly, although the anesthesia is "local" the

drugs are absorbed into the circulation just as with any injectable medication so that a generalized effect also occurs. Local anesthetic agents produce side effects on the heart, blood vessels, and brain. Overdosage can lead to serious consequences such as dangerous heart rhythms or convulsions. Allergies and idiosyncracies can also produce fatal collapse in sensitive patients. Thus, even the simplist anesthetic agents can cause dangerous side effects.

Nevertheless, properly used, local is the safest form of chemical anesthesia and probably should be used more frequently in favor of more risky techniques. With careful, use, local anesthesia can even be used for major operations. Japanese surgeons have developed methods for using local anesthetic to include even extensive stomach and bowel resections.

In this country, surgeons sometimes use local for major operations for patients who are elderly or debilitated and might not tolerate more risky techniques. Furthermore, many operations traditionally done with general anesthesia, such as hernia repair and breast operations, can readily be accomplished under local. But some surgeons are not familiar with the techniques or do not want to be hampered by repeat injections or alert, responsive patients. Unaware of the increased risks, some anxious patients also prefer to be asleep during operations.

Regional anesthesia is a broader form of "local," in which the drugs are injected directly around large major nerves. For instance, carefully injected *caine* drugs around the three major nerves near the shoulder can give excellent anesthesia to the entire arm and hand for up to an hour and a half. Similarly, nerve trunks to the legs or ankles can be blocked. But with regional anesthesia additional risks become important. Injury to major arteries and veins or organs such as the bladder or lungs can occur. Also, permanant nerve damage has resulted from this technique. Because the difficulty of making exacting injections results in unreliability and risks, regional anesthesia is not used extensively.

Spinal anesthesia may be thought of as a regional block applied to the main nerve of the body, the spinal cord itself. Following injection of *caine* derivatives into the space surrounding the spinal cord, anesthesia and temporary paralysis is produced from that point downward in the body. The technique is relatively easy and provides reliable and effective anesthesia for an hour and a half or so. The needle injection into the spine is uncomfortable but tolerable. The most frequent complication, spinal headache, is not serious but can be extremely uncomfortable for a few days.

Though often discussed, permanent paralysis of the lower extremities following spinal anesthesia is extremely rare. More serious complications usually result from sudden drops in blood pressure, which occur frequently. Heart attacks and brain and kidney damage can result from the shock of lowered blood pressure during spinal anesthesia. Careful monitoring of vital signs is essential to prevent these complications.

Epidural or *caudal* is a special type of spinal anesthesia used for procedures around the pelvis. It has proved especially useful during childbirth. With caudal anesthesia, the *caine* derivatives are slowly dripped into a space around the spinal cord, allowing for minute-to-minute control for hours. Paralysis does not occur and the birth process can continue normally. One disadvantage to caudal is the requirement of constant monitoring, which is inconvenient for doctors and hospital staffs. The technique also carries with it all the complications of spinal anesthetic.

General anesthesia is the most extensively used form of pain relief during operations. Anesthesia is produced by medications that are injected into veins or that are absorbed from their gaseous state through the lungs and into the circulation. The medications profoundly affect the entire body.

With general anesthesia, patients are not only paralyzed but are rendered unconscious as well. All bodily functions are impaired, and heartbeat, breathing, and blood pressure all must be attended to by the anesthesiologist. Even hormonal balances are interrupted by general anesthesia.

The vital organs are all affected by these side effects, and any of the serious complications we have mentioned can happen at any time. So complex is the administration of general anesthesia that doctors say, " . . . if you think everything is going along smoothly, you must be missing something."

Nondrug Anesthesia

In search of ideal anesthetics, doctors and others have turned to nondrug techniques that use mental abilities or unknown neurological phenomena to achieve pain control. The LaMaze breathing technique for the pain of childbirth has been widely accepted. This technique has also been shown to be effective for postoperative pain, but because it requires additional patient care in the recovery room and wards it has not come into widespread use.

Before the advent of modern anesthesia, more unusual methods were occasionally tried. One famous nineteenth-century surgeon, Guilliarme Dupuytren, who was known for his contemptuousness, actually induced a fainting spell in a woman patient by making a brutal remark. During the ensuing brief period of anesthesia, he quickly and painlessly lanced the woman's abscess.

Hypnosis for relief of pain has been attempted ever since Mesmer popularized the techniques in the eighteenth century. Because of the mysticism and charlatantry associated with hypnotism through the centuries, however, the medical profession has not embraced this form of anesthesia. Nevertheless, the remarkable demonstrations of individuals being rendered free of pain on stages or in nightclubs tantalized doctors to try the techniques in operating rooms.

The phenomenon of hypnotism is undeniable and one wonders why it is not used more in surgery. Reports indicate that under conditions of research, only about 20 percent of patients respond satisfactorily to hypnosis for pain relief. That number could undoubtedly be improved with more practice and research if hypnosis received high priority within the medical profession. Though hypnosis seems ideal, because it would free anesthesia from the serious side effects of drugs, it is time-consuming and therefore impractical in our busy operating rooms. Still, qualified hypnotists are available in most communities and even a few anesthesiologists have shown some interest.

Acupuncture, another alternate form of anesthesia, has received much publicity recently. Pictures from China showing wide-awake patients undergoing major surgery painlessly with only a few needles in place have been in newspapers and magazines. But acupuncture has not been carefully studied and developed in the Western world, and though it can be remarkably effective for some patients, it also suffers from unreliability and cumbersomeness. The fact that it works at all, is fascinating and warrants further investigation. But, like hypnosis, acupuncture has not enjoyed widespread interest from doctors. One can only speculate about how efficacious these safe modes of anesthesia might become if they commanded more interest from the public and more research and development by medical professionals.

Now that you know about the different types of anesthesia and some of the dangers involved, you can proceed to learn all you can about your own case, if and when the time comes. You will be able to face your operation more confidently if you observe the following precautions:

1) Avoid unnecessary surgery—in that way you will also avoid the risks of anesthesia.
2) Ask for and accept the safest anesthesia that will give you adequate freedom from pain. Think about the risks of anesthesia and decide whether a little discomfort isn't worth avoiding significant risks.
3) Learn all you can about your anesthesia and your anesthetist beforehand. Make the most of the preoperative visit to help to relieve your fears and apprehensions.
4) If you want to try alternative modes of anesthesia, such as hypnotism or acupuncture, make plans well ahead of time. You can probably find such help if you want it.
5) Never accept anesthesia from anyone who has not thoroughly evaluated your case and your medical history ahead of time or who does not instill confidence in you.

8

Surgery—I Need It?

———————————•———————————

Minor surgery:
An operation performed upon someone else.

Imagine yourself being advised to have an operation. The nurse ushers you into the doctor's private consultation room. It's not the brightly lit clinical examining room where you were seen before. This time it's the inner sanctum, the carefully appointed office with subdued wallpaper, soft lights, and shelves of books—lots of books. You look up from the overstuffed chair and see a conspicuous display of diplomas and credentials on the wall, each framed document attesting to the doctor's learned wisdom.

Soon, the surgeon steps into the room. He sits down in the leather swivel chair behind his huge mahogany desk and removes his glasses, rubbing his eyes as if to relieve his fatigue. As he begins to speak, his eyes remain noncommital, and he neither smiles nor frowns. Instead, his expression is emotionless, not revealing any personal anxiety about the pronouncement he is about to make.

In carefully measured phrases, the doctor methodically explains that after thorough evaluation of your symptoms and examinations, and after review of your X rays and laboratory test, your diagnosis dictates that major surgery be performed to remove the disease from your body—and the sooner the better.

What will you think? Will you immediately believe the doctor? How will you feel? Will you be afraid? What will you do? Will you jump from the chair and run out the door, or will you control your fears and try objectively to study the advice? Will you try to appear brave, then go home to lie awake at night in fear? To whom will you turn for guidance or help? What will you say?

Obviously, you would be able to face such a confrontation more comfortable and confidently if you prepared yourself ahead of time. Whether the advice to have an operation might come to you in a doctor's office, an emergency room, or a clinic, you should plan ahead or else when the time comes you may have little choice except to accept the doctor's seemingly expert advice and proceed with the necessary arrangements, reporting to the hospital as instructed and following directions like a good patient.

If you do that, you will eventually be put flat on your back on a stretcher, wheeled into an operating room, and have inflicted upon you an operation the necessity of which you will never know, the nature of which you will be unsure, and the potentially disasterous risks of which you will be completely unaware.

Afterward, you will awaken in a recovery room, alone and in severe pain, still facing the suffering of recovery and the possibility of terrifying complications, even death.

If, on the other hand, you wish to assume some personal responsibility for your case and to have more to say about what is going to happen, you are already prepared to begin. You know that although surgery can be truly beneficial, it is an inexact science and that doctors frequently disagree about modes of therapy.

You know that competence and ethics vary among surgeons, and that excessive scientific zeal, advocacy for the surgical approach to disease, and the selfish motivations of the private practice of surgery as a profit-making business are elements that actually work against you.

You have also learned that all surgery is fraught with complications and that the risks of any operation must be weighed against potential benefits.

Furthermore, you are now aware that frequently medical alternatives might enable you to avoid the risks of an operation. Most importantly, you know that you have a right to all the facts about a proposed operation and that surgeons are legally required not only to answer all your questions but to offer voluntarily all substantive information about your treatment.

Indeed, your evaluation and decision-making process about surgery can begin even as you sit in that chair in the surgeon's consultation room. Instead of becoming anxious and fearfully succumbing to the recommendation, you can remain calm, recognizing that his advice is only one man's opinion, and that you have a series of steps to go through before accepting. To begin with, you already know that unless the operation is an immediate lifesaving emergency or a severe emergency, you have time to think about it. So you won't rush, and you won't let anyone rush you. Remember, there are no such things as stupid questions—there are only stupid answers. So, start asking questions—lots of questions.

You should remember that doctors are accustomed to being treated as experts, if not deities. Consequently, they are not usually asked more than a few superficial questions about treatment, especially proposed surgery. Therefore, you might be wise not to pose your queries in an accusative or suspicious manner, suggesting that you don't trust the doctor or that you question his medical knowledge or judgment. If you express your questions as genuine concerns and indicate a sincere desire to learn more about illness and treatment, those doctors who are confident of their own abilities will receive them well. One surgeon even collected reprints from the medical literature and made a housecall to discuss the entire case with a family who had expressed particular concern. Become suspicious if you ask questions in an honest and appreciative manner and the surgeon seems evasive or irritated. Perhaps that doctor really doesn't know the answers to your questions. Perhaps he lacks the knowledge and the self-confidence to respond graciously.

From reading this book you know what questions to ask. For instance, remembering the inexactitudes in surgical practice, you will ask the doctor *how* he came to his conclusion. You will ask him about the probabilities that his diagnosis is correct and that the proposed operation might work. What is the statistical risk of serious complications, including death? How would the surgeon candidly weigh the potential benefits versus the possible harm? Are there various choices of operations, some more radical and risky than others? Is there anything in your particular case that might lead to a different outcome? Could there possibly be a change in plan during the operation? Finally, you should ask what the alternatives to the operation are. This might be a difficult area of discussion because, as you know, surgeons believe in their skills and tend to consider medical alternatives as inferior or lesser modalities. Nevertheless, you should persist until you know what the alternatives are.

Don't be afraid to ask the surgeon about himself. Ask him where he trained, what his qualifications are, and how long he has been in practice. If he answers that he trained "back east" or "in California," ask him to be more specific. Ask him how many times he has performed the operation he proposes for you.

Obviously, talking to a doctor about his qualifications can be a delicate matter. However, questions asked in an honest and friendly manner, indicating an effort to get to know the doctor, should not be a problem. It's reasonable for you to want to get to know someone who is literally going to take you life into his hands. Besides, most excellent surgeons don't mind such questioning at all. It gives them a chance to proclaim openly their competence and thus gain your confidence.

For you, it may be the best oppotunity to evaluate the surgeon for yourself. Observe how readily he answers your questions and how willing he is to be open about himself and his training. His relative candor and forthrightness may tell you a great deal about his character. If you like the surgeon, keep him in mind until you have more thoroughly evaluated your illness as well as some other surgeons. If you don't like the surgeon, then *please,* leave his office and find someone else. Trust your instincts. Aside from the doctor's competence, the last thing you need in an operation is a surgeon whom you dislike.

Evaluating surgeons is not easy, and you will have to use every method available. One potential source of information is other doctors. They usually know about surgeons because they have the opportunity of seeing their colleagues in action. In fact, almost every doctor has a firm idea of which one or two surgeons in the world he would allow to operate upon himself or his family. Unfortunately, you probably couldn't get doctors to tell you who these choices would be.

Even though it's perfectly ethical for you to ask about the competence of surgeons, it seems that, ironically, doctors consider it unethical to give you an honest answer. When asking other doctors about a particular surgeon, you may learn more from what they do not say than from what they do say. Remember, the business, professional, and social interactions among doctors is very complex and you may have great difficulty finding an unbiased opinion. But surgeons are not gods, and you can trust your feelings about them just as you can intuitively evaluate anyone.

Probably the best way for you to choose a surgeon is simply to talk to him personally about your illness and the proposed treatment, and about himself, and then decide for yourself on the basis of his training and experience, his helpfulness and his candor.

Getting a Second Opinion

After evaluating the recommendation for surgery and the doctor who gave it, you are ready for other opinions. In the process you can evaluate other surgeons. If you are going to ask other surgeons for second opinions about your case, certain precautions are in order.

First, try to avoid the tendency to place too much credence upon what the second surgeon says. Remember, he is just as likely to be wrong as the first. Second, be careful whom you choose. Surgeons in the same practice, in the same hospital, or even in the same community are often reluctant to disagree with one another, and under such circumstances you will receive only a rubber-stamp approval instead of a carefully considered opinion.

But it's more compelling than that. Think of the position of the second surgeon. Even if he doesn't openly admit the limitations of his so-called science, he intuitively knows that his decisions rest almost solely upon judgment—often little more than educated guesses. During his training and practice he has seen older surgeons in positions of authority criticize and contradict younger men only to be dead wrong later.

Think, for instance, of a surgeon being asked for a second opinion about a recommendation for appendectomy. He knows that the diagnosis is difficult, fraught with a 25 percent margin of error. What if he contradicts the first surgeon and then is shown to be wrong when the appendix ruptures and the patient goes into septic shock? The responsibility for such a decision is almost too much to ask—and the legal implications frightening. Indeed, except in cases of flagrant misrepresentation, giving a contradictory second opinion takes courage—which some would say borders on foolhardiness. How much more comfortable just to go along with the first surgeon, leaving the responsibility to him.

But the whole process can work in reverse, also, especially for surgeons with many friends in the medical power structure. One young surgeon remembers that during his first five years of practice in a very competitive suburban community, there was not one single second-opinion consultation in which any of the older surgeons agreed with him. How could that be? Is medical and surgical science really so inexact that a competent young surgeon would constantly disagree with his colleagues? Certainly not. The fact was that in that community there were far too many surgeons and the competition for patients was keen. So, when the established surgeons gave second opinions they always disagreed. That way they could steal the cases, perform the operations, and collect the fees. Often they frightened patients into immediate operations; in other cases, they postponed operations for further evaluation. Either way, they could get the case and the fee for themselves.

If you are planning to get a second opinion, seek a surgeon who does not know the surgeon who gave you the first opinion, or at least one who does not practice in the same hospital. To ensure an unbiased opinion, I suggest you find a surgeon in another neighborhood, even from another city or county.

When you stop to think about it, finding a valid second opinion is no easier than obtaining a trustworthy first opinion. If you are lucky enough to have close friends or relatives who are physicians, you may have a good source—at least, they might look out for your best interests. University hospitals have traditionally been a good source for second opinions because they are outside the competitive mainstream of day-to-day surgical business practices. Unfortunately, however, most university professors have taken up part-time private practices to augment their incomes. Obviously, in doing so they also become suspect of bias on account of the quest for business profits.

Perhaps the best second opinions would come from internists who specialize in the area of your particular illness. Most good internists are familiar with the operative indications for diseases in their own field. More importantly, they are almost always more conservative than their surgical counterparts because they do not derive personal gain from surgical fees. But beware of internists bearing gadgets—catheters, scopes, and probes with which to perform special X rays or diagnostic tests. While using such equipment, these otherwise noninvasive specialists become similar to surgeons, performing operations for fees.

Remember, all those coronary bypass patients are supplied to the thoracic surgeons by cardiologists, who themselves collect large fees for the diagnostic cardiac catheterization, and for monitoring the patients during surgery. Beware also of exasperated internists. Sometimes when a patient does not respond satisfactorily to treatment, the family doctor or internist becomes frustrated, especially when patients or their families show excessive concern. Obvious solution—send the patient to a surgeon. Most good surgeons occasionally find themselves pushed to operate upon patients who might be better off without surgery. Nevertheless, if you consult a heart specialist, a gastroenterologist, a kidney specialist, or whatever internist is appropriate to your case, you might be surprised to learn the many alternatives to surgery available to you.

There are some alternatives that you are unlikely to learn about from physicians. These are forms of therapy which are especially appropriate for illnesses with psychosomatic components. I am referring to personal, inner experiences, such as transcendental meditation and yoga, which date back thousands of years and were considered perfectly natural forms of self-help and enhancement. With the advent of modern medicine, these techniques were discarded because they were not considered to be scientific enough. Recognizing their potential, however, is a movement known as holistic medicine, which attempts to revive them, and through new applications in the form of biofeedback and directive behavioral therapy, many patients have found relief of such ailments as headache, arthritis, neurological problems, and high blood pressure.

Surgeons often recommend operations for emotionally involved ailments, such as peptic ulcer disease, when standard medical therapy fails. But the potential benefits of holistic medicine upon such diseases have not been adequately studied. There is good reason to believe that many diseases now treated surgically might respond to holistic approaches. Depending upon individual preferences, of course, some patients with ulcers, ulcerative colitis, high blood pressure, even heart disease, might benefit from a trial of holistic medicine rather than immediately submitting to the risks of surgery.

When all is said and done, perhaps you should think of second opinions only as sources of information to help you compare different modes of therapy and different surgeons. In the final analysis, there is little doubt that if you want to be careful, the decisions for you and your family must come from you. If you learn what this book has to offer and then study your illness and proposed operation, you will be the best person in the world to give the final opinion. All you have to do is follow some simple steps:

1) Stay calm. Remember that a recommendation for surgery is just one doctor's opinion until you learn more.

2) Take your time. You will have a lot to learn, but unless your case is an immediate lifesaving or severe emergency you have time to think and discuss the case with other doctors, family, and friends.

3) Read this book again and read about your operation in Chapter Fourteen.

4) Ask questions—many questions. Become *informed.*

5) Ask your doctors specifically what the indications are for surgery—including the statistical figures that point to an operation in your case.

6) Ask about the potential benefits and the chances that the operation will result in same.

7) Ask about possible risks, complications, and side effects.

Do not be afraid to discuss unpleasant possibilities such as loss of limb or death.

8) Evaluate your surgeon by asking about his training and experience and by carefully observing his answers. Use your intuition and your ability to judge others' personalities to come to a decision about who you want to be your surgeon.

9) Get additional opinions.

10) Decide about all alternative modes of treatment.

11) Talk it over with family and friends and apply some good common sense in addition to the medical jargon.

12) Decide whether to have the proposed surgery. Remember, *it's your decision.*

After you have decided that an operation would be the best treatment for you and have selected a surgeon, you should give some thought as to who will be the assistant surgeon in your case. Most people never think about that and leave the decision to their doctors. However, it is a point you should consider in terms of the quality and safety of your operation. After all, the assistant surgeon will receive a fee amounting to approximately twenty percent of the surgeon's charge! And he has no responsibility for your diagnosis or your postoperative care. But what does he do for that fee?

One male nurse was allowed to observe a brain operation on his uncle. He noticed that the assistant surgeon (the family doctor who was unqualified to perform surgery) merely stood by and observed except at one point when the surgeon said, "Pass the suction." The assistant reached to the instrument table and handed the suction to the surgeon. For that, the family was charged $400.

Regardless of their qualifications, many assistant surgeons in the United States are family doctors or other practitioners who referred the case to the surgeon in the first place. In this modern version of fee splitting, many doctors tacitly agree that the referring physician gets to assist at the surgery in order to gain the nice fee. Some surgeons advocate that for the safety of the patient only board-certified specialists or surgical residents in training be allowed to assist during surgery. After all, there is an abundance of surgeons who are more than willing to assist. But in the competitive business of surgery, surgeons can't afford to offend their referral sources, so the use of unqualified assistants goes on.

Wouldn't you like to have an assistant for your operation who is himself a skilled surgeon, and can provide not only expert technical help but also consultation for any problems that might arise? Furthermore, what about the rare possibility that your surgeon might become ill or otherwise incapacitated during your operation? Wouldn't you like to have someone there competent to take over? If so, you should ask about who will assist at your operation. You may have to insist on a certified surgeon.

Finally, you are ready to prepare for your operation. The following chapters will tell you how you can prepare psychologically and physically for entering the hospital, undergoing the operations, and recuperating. You will learn how you can take charge of your case to help prevent complications or problems and to speed your own return to good health.

9
Getting Ready
for the Big Day

———•———

*A journey of a thousand miles begins with one
step.*

Lao-tse

You have decided that surgery is necessary. You were advised
by your doctor that an operation was indicated to treat hemorrhoids, hernias, stones, inflammation, ulcers, bumps, lumps,
tumors, or whatever might be the problem in your particular
case. After that, you asked many, many questions and obtained
additional opinions. You found out all the important factors
about the proposed surgery—the operation, surgeon, diagnosis,
indications, alternatives, anesthesia, potential benefits, and possible complications. Then you weighed the benefits against the
risks and decided to have the operation.

Your surgeon scheduled you for admission to the hospital
and reserved a place for you on the operating room schedule.
But what did he tell you to do in the meantime? Were all your
questions answered and a full program of preparation outlined
for you? Aside from specific medications or treatments, did
your surgeon explain what you might do personally to prepare
for surgery? Aside from telling you to quit smoking and get
plenty of rest, did he mention anything you could do to prevent
problems in your case? If not, don't be too surprised. After all,
you should know by now from having read thus far that we
surgeons train in hospital-based and disease-oriented programs
with very little attention paid to preventive medicine. Even our

textbooks and the American College of Surgeons' manual of preoperative care concentrate almost exclusively on in-hospital care.

As you left your surgeon's office, you may have felt an ominous twinge inside when he said, "Try not to worry." If you're like most people, you *will* worry. You will be distracted during the day and unable to sleep at night, wondering about your illness and the risk of the operation. You may feel helpless and wish there was something you could do besides just wait . . . and wait. Well, take heart. Unless your case is a severe emergency, you can do many important things to get ready. In fact, even considering all the medical knowledge of your doctors and nurses and the scientific facilities from which you might benefit, what you do for yourself may make the difference of whether you suffer complications—even whether you live or die.

We can't talk about improving your health without discussing some of the activities you should give up. If you really want to help yourself through surgery, you just cannot deny the desirability of kicking those habits you know to be harmful to you. Excessive smoking, alcohol, and coffee all have directly adverse effects upon your ability to tolerate surgery.

Smoking causes an irritative bronchitis that in turn leads to decreased pulmonary function and predisposes you to lung collapse and pneumonia. Furthermore, the nicotine in tobacco has profound deleterious effects upon heart function. Alcohol also impairs heart function and inhibits the liver processes so dearly needed for protein metabolism and healing. Caffeine profoundly impairs your heart and circulation. Together or separately, they all decrease your resistance to complications. You simply cannot undergo an operation optimally if you persist in these harmful habits.

You already know that your operation will inflict a profound physiological insult upon your body and that complications seem to be just waiting for the opportunity to attack. You know that you depend upon your body's natural defenses to ward off or combat the ravages of human error, drug reactions, nonhealing, hemorrhage, and infection. If your resistance is low, you are weakened by illness; if you are in less than optimal health, you will be far more susceptible. If, by chance, you happen to be a health enthusiast and keep yourself in perfect condition, you may feel ready for your operation. Chances are, however, that there is room for improvement of some specific factors of which you are unaware and for which you are not prepared.

On the other hand, if, like most people, you don't exercise enough, pay little attention to proper nutrition, are overweight, fail to get proper rest, overwork and overplay, and abuse your body with caffeine, nicotine, alcohol, and perhaps even some other prescribed or self-administered drugs, preparing for your operation may mean nothing less than a drastic change in your way of life.

Start Emotionally

What can you do? Well, entire textbooks have been devoted to scientific preoperative evaluation and preparation. But that kind of information demands intensive study and may well be better left to your surgeon. If you have asked questions, you will already know the medical facts that pertain to your case. If you have chosen your surgeon carefully, and if he's board-certified, that's just the kind of thing he should be really good at. But chances are your surgeon is not very knowledgeable about other important facets of preoperative health care, which do not appear in the textbooks—psychological, nutritional, and exercise needs.

Regardless of your state of health, your emotional adjustment to surgery is one of the most important facets of your preparation. Certainly, you can expect to be emotionally upset before major surgery. In the face of a threatening operation, anxiety is perfectly normal. However, excessive emotional turmoil can become almost unbearable when the fear of the unknown and feelings of helplessness become superimposed upon underlying emotional problems or the stresses of work, family, or personal life situations.

Most patients will have to find ways to relieve that anxiety. Freedom from severe anxiety can mean less chance of developing psychological complications after surgery. The study mentioned earlier in which women showed significantly less anxiety and greater contentment after becoming thoroughly informed about hysterectomy is only one example.

Children given puppet therapy and motion picture preparation for surgery were observed to have significantly fewer emotional disturbances both before and after their operations. Even patients undergoing open-heart surgery have decreased incidence of postoperative mental aberrations when counseled beforehand. But lowering anxiety can have important salutary physical effects, too.

In one study, patients who were counseled about postoperative nausea had significantly less vomiting after their operations than control subjects. In another study, patients who experienced lowered anxiety levels preoperatively required fewer barbiturates and other anesthetic agents during their operations, significantly reducing their risk of serious or lethal complications from drugs. Indeed, some authors have pointed out that by decreasing physical risks, lowered anxiety can actually save patients' lives.

There can be little doubt that lowering your anxiety before surgery can result in immeasurable emotional and physical benefits. Yet, with our efficient, technological approach to modern surgery, the emotional needs of patients are all too often neglected. The ambience of surgical wards and operating rooms—the mysterious activities of busy doctors and nurses, the dripping of fluids in plastic tubing, the whirring and beeping of futuristic electronic devices—is enough to test the nerves of even the most well-adjusted individuals. Not only that, the usual medical approaches for the relief of anxiety are all too often ineffective.

As I have pointed out, surgeons are not trained in emotional counseling. Besides, they are often too busy and preoccupied with the many demanding aspects of scientific surgical care to offer more than brief counseling. Even when offered, the advice usually implies that you should trust the doctors and the miracles of modern medicine to see you through.

Although such cursory attempts at supportive therapy may help some patients, closer scrutiny has shown that it actually increases anxiety in most patients. For extreme cases, surgeons might obtain psychiatric consultations. But for most, the next line of therapeutics is usually tranquilizers. In our drug-oriented medical system, tranquilizers attempt to provide easy solutions to emotional problems that would require time-consuming personal involvement. In hospitals, these drugs also offer solutions to the logistics problems of wheeling patients into operating rooms, getting the job done, and moving them back down hallways to their rooms. In that atmosphere, anxious, emotionally troubled patients all too often are seen as uncooperative troublemakers, obstructing the doctors' and nurses' unfailing dedication to curing diseases and distracting them from a higher sense of duty.

Certain lucky patients might happen to find solace from a nurse willing to take time from her coffee break. A few patients might be comforted by a perceptive nurses' aide, a medical student, or a volunteer worker. On occasion, even a surgeon might find his way to his almost forgotten feelings of compassion. Most patients, however, will simply be given tranquilizers, and thus be unnecessarily exposed to their dangerous, even lethal side effects.

Ironically, most of the patients will not obtain relief of their anxieties with drugs. Careful studies have shown that patients given tranquilizers prior to operations were sedated, but still measured higher anxiety levels than patients who were counseled instead of being given medications. Once again, a closer look shows that medical technology and drugs are no substitute for human understanding.

When facing surgery, you may therefore need to find ways to relieve anxiety for yourself. That is one of the reasons I have stressed the importance of becoming informed about your operation beforehand. Coming to a personal decision about surgery and having more to say about what is going to happen are in themselves factors that can lower your anxiety by giving you more of a sense of control over your own destiny. But there are other ways for you to cope with the anxiety and fears normally associated with surgery.

Perhaps the most important way is to talk about your fears and apprehensions with those you can trust. An understanding doctor can be of immeasurable benefit, but close friends and loved ones are equally important. Some people might find reassurance through religious counseling, others will need help from social workers, psychologists, or psychiatrists.

Through the deep experiences found with meditation and yoga many people have not only found ways to cope with stress but have gone on to experience richer and more fulfilling lives. Earlier, I suggested these modes of therapy as possible alternatives to surgery for the treatment of psychosomatic disorders. They are also particularly suitable for relieving preoperative anxiety because the common benefit from all forms of meditation is the alleviation of stress responses to threatening stimuli.

Furthermore, research has shown that people who meditate become more psychologically stable, less anxious, and seem to develop an inner sense of effectiveness rather than submitting to stress as passive victims of circumstance. What could be more tailor-made for helping preoperative anxiety? Indeed, if you have ever considered trying one of these methods of self-enhancement, perhaps now, before your operation, is the time to begin. It's really quite easy to get started. You don't have to join a quasi-religious group or human potential movement to make meditation work for you. Bookstores and libraries have many good references, and holistic clinics and individuals are readily available to help you with most types of Zen, transcendental meditation, and yoga.

Health and Nutrition

Nutrition is another important aspect of preparation for your operation. You know that an operation places metabolic demands upon your body, and that a good diet is essential for normal healing and to defend against complications.

Of course, you may think that because you eat three meals a day regularly, that you're a healthy, all-American specimen. You may believe that being just a little overweight, doesn't mean you have poor nutrition. Well, don't be so sure. Many nutritionists say that the image of the well-nourished American is a myth.

Experts estimate that as many as 80 percent of people in the United States are malnourished—and that includes the obese.

National surveys show that most people have low levels of one or more essential nutrients. In one experiment, even rats failed to grow or thrive normally on the equivalent of the average American diet. Moreover, some nutritionists believe that many illnesses can be linked to poor nutrition and estimate a 25 percent reduction in infections, respiratory and cardiac disease with improved diet. As you contemplate surgery, perhaps you should think more about your nutrition.

Don't expect a great deal of help from your surgeon. When he recommended surgery, did he talk to you about nutrition? Probably not. Most surgeons do not fully appreciate that nutrition is an essential part of good practice and rarely advise patients about dietary needs. Only 25 percent of American medical schools offer specific courses in nutrition, and most surgical textbooks mention nutrition only in terms of particular diseases and therapeutic intravenous feedings. One reputable textbook simply states that the average surgical patient needs only a normal American diet. Even the *Manual of Surgical Nutrition* published by the American College of Surgeons refers to surgical nutrition only for patients in hospitals.

As a matter of fact, most surgeons couldn't tell you the basic nutritional requirements for health, let alone for diseased states or periods of recovery. Surgeons seem to be more interested in how long patients can live without food than with what constitutes good health. Yet, in a careful study, 83 percent of patients admitted to a hospital were found to have one vitamin deficiency; 68 percent had two or more. In another survey, experts found that patients were operated upon without adequate nutritional care either before or afterward. More ominously, in one hospital, of twenty patients whose surgical wounds failed to heal, all were found to have below normal proteins and nineteen had vitamin deficiencies.

You can help prepare yourself for surgery in many ways. First, if you are overweight, you should shed some of that excess fat bulging around your waistline. It is a form of malnutrition. All that extra tissue is a burden on your system. It reduces the freedom with which you move, impairs your circulation, decreases expansion of your lungs, and places greater demands upon your cardiac function. The additional stress of surgery, especially if complications set in, may be just too much for your system. Not only that, fat is a deterrent to wound healing because it creates more tension on the sutures, causes more oozing of blood, and increases swelling. Losing weight before surgery is not easy because you must maintain adequate nutritional requirements for healing and recovery while lowering caloric intake. But it can be done. Certainly, you should work with your doctor or a nutritionist, but it is possible to eat adequate protein, vitamins, and minerals and still lose excess weight prior to surgery.

Understanding nutrition requires some effort. Concepts in normal requirements have changed in the past few years as more and more people have become aware of the effects of food materials on bodily and mental function. Standards of minimum daily requirements have been questioned, the use of large doses of vitamins for the prevention of diseases has been advocated, and previously unknown functions of vitamins upon brain function have been elucidated. Older concepts of the relationships of fats, carbohydrates, and proteins have been put aside in favor of newer methods of maintaining proper nutrition. The role of trace elements such as zinc, selenium, sulfur, magnesium, and chromium have been discovered. But nutrition doesn't have to be all that complicated. You could learn about your own basic food requirements in a few hours with a good book on the subject.

One of the first aspects of nutrition to be discovered was the importance of protein for normal healing. The observation was made when laboratory research animals failed to heal properly. Later, more careful studies showed that large amounts of protein are lost in the urine of patients for approximately ten days following surgery. The reason for this negative nitrogen balance is not altogether clear, but because of it, protein requirements following surgery increase to three times normal. The effect of protein losses are compounded because patients usually cannot eat before and after surgery.

Although most patients seem to tolerate the protein loss, little is known about why others suffer from healing problems or suffer complications for no apparent reason. Although surgeons have developed methods for giving intravenous protein to patients on prolonged starvation or with complicated illnesses or obvious deficiencies, little attention is paid to the average patient until problems develop. In fact, most surgeons are quick to point out that there is no scientific evidence that increasing protein preoperatively enhances wound healing. But are there unmeasured or unknown protein deficiencies in patients who do not recover from operations normally? The research has not been done. To complete a statistically significant study would require thousands of patients and many years.

Carbohydrates and fats are important in surgery only insofar as they affect general health and because of the possibility they might spare some protein losses. As you have probably heard, however, most Americans eat too much of these foodstuffs and should find ways to balance their diets for optimal health.

How Vitamins Help

Most people know about vitamins—the established minimum daily requirements are listed on the back of cereal boxes and health tonics. We know that gross vitamin deficiencies cause serious diseases, such as beriberi, pellagra, scurvy, and rickets, but we do not know about the possible role of undetectable or periodic vitamin inadequacies, or whether increased vitamin intake could help prevent disease. Some nutritionists contend that the accepted daily requirements may actually be below what would be optimal for health.

Additionally, we know that requirements for vitamins increase dramatically during illness and surgery. For instance, Vitamin A is essential for the formation of the protein networks for healing wounds. Experimental animals healed significantly faster and with stronger scars when given Vitamin A supplements. Other studies showed that Vitamin A supplements can prevent such complications as postoperative stress ulcers of the stomach.

The daily requirements of B vitamins also increases to as much as twenty times normal under conditions of illness or surgery. These important B vitamins act as catalysts for metabolic processes which utilize nutrients to build new protein for wound healing. Furthermore, they are essential for the normal function of the heart, liver, brain, adrenal glands, and blood cells. Virtually every organ of the body needs B vitamins to combat the possible stress of surgery.

The requirements for Vitamin C also increase during surgery. Indeed, Vitamin C has been called *the surgeons' vitamin* because it is an essential component in forming scar tissue. Deficiencies cause marked delays in wound healing. But postoperative infections also require increased Vitamin C. In one study of over fourteen hundred patients with surgical infections, all were found to have Vitamin C levels as low as in patients with scurvy. The effects of large doses of Vitamin C to prevent the common cold has led to speculation about its possible use in preventing other infections.

Vitamin D is especially important in orthopedic surgery for healing of fractures or bone operations. The full effects of Vitamin E are unknown, but it is involved in connective tissue diseases and may be required for proper scar formation. Vitamin K is of special interest because of its effect upon the liver for forming blood-clotting factors essential in the prevention of hemorrhage.

Many minerals have special importance to surgery, the most notable of which is iron. Not only does iron play an important role in muscle function and wound healing, but it is integral to oxygen transport so essential for heart and lung function. For surgical patients, increased iron intake is important to replace deficiencies caused by not eating and by losses due to bleeding during operations.

Recently, zinc has been found to have a profound effect upon postoperative wound healing. This element is involved in the synthesis of DNA, a special protein that functions with the cells themselves. In one study, scar tissue was healthier and stronger in patients given supplemental zinc. In another study, women given 150 milligrams of zinc a day required significantly shorter hospitalizations postoperatively than women receiving ordinary hospital diets.

The whole subject of nutrition requires more than can be discussed here. However, just eating a normal American diet is no guarantee that you will have adequate nutrition, and your requirements for proteins, vitamins, and minerals increase dramatically during and following surgery. Furthermore, with most patients, surgeons take nutrition for granted, and your nutritional state will not likely be evaluated before your operation. Perhaps you should take charge of your nutrition for yourself. It could make the difference of whether your operation goes smoothly or becomes complicated. Books about nutrition are readily available.

Exercise

In recent years, exercise has become recognized as an important part of recuperation from surgery. In fact, the initiation of early ambulation rather than strict bed rest after surgery may have done more to decrease postoperative mortality than any other advance in the past hundred years.

Additionally, deep-breathing and coughing exercises are known to be highly beneficial to lung function and to prevent lung collapse and pneumonia. But what about new trends in exercise—jogging, dance, and aerobics? These have been shown to be highly beneficial for bodily function and well-being. Although these exercises have not been adopted as a routine part of preoperative preparation, there is little question that they would be of immeasurable benefit.

Exercising gives the exact improvement in bodily function that is most desirable for improving patients' ability to withstand the stresses of surgery and to avoid complications. Increased utilization of oxygen, improved heart efficiency, increased cardiorespiratory reserve, and markedly improved circulation are just what the doctor ordered for surgical patients.

In fact, techniques and equipment have been developed for use in hospitals to improve these functions for patients with heart or lung disease. But these innovations can give only a fraction of the beneficial results you can obtain for yourself by simply exercising adequately.

Of course, you may have to consult your doctor as to whether exercise is safe considering your illness. But in most cases any harmful possibilities would be far outweighed by the immense advantages—a dramatic improvement in your resistance to circulatory, lung, heart, and infectious complications. If you don't know how to begin, ask an expert at a health spa or get a book on the subject. Perhaps you've thought for a long time about exercising more. There could be no better time to start.

Many surgeons do not recommend these methods of preparation for operations. They point out that there is no scientific evidence to demonstrate that meditation, nutritional programs, or exercise improve your chances for surviving an operation. But perhaps you'll forgive us surgeons. You see, we were trained to think of disease and not of preventive medicine.

Not only that, as persons purporting to be scientific, we cannot endorse treatment that is not supported by statistics. Our godlike posture does not allow us to recommend programs which have not been more or less proved. Furthermore, if we talked about transcendental meditation, health food, or jogging at a scientific meeting about preoperative care, we would be ridiculed by our colleagues. If we persisted, we might even risk being formally censured by the medical society, or even worse, sued by patients who become dissatisfied. Can you imagine a doctor in a courtroom under cross-examination trying to defend his prescription for yoga or Zen?

So, perhaps I should clarify right now that I'm not directly recommending these health measures. You can decide for yourself if they're important. You know that lowering your anxiety will help you through your operation. You know that proper nutrition can greatly improve your healing powers. You know that exercise will help you withstand potential complications of surgery. But if you're like most people, you have thought many times about improving your lifestyle and quitting some of your bad habits. You may have even considered enhancing yourself mentally, improving your diet, and beginning to exercise. But there always seemed to be plenty of time to worry about those things *later*. The detrimental effects weren't likely to become apparent for years. But the time is up. Facing an operation, the potential deleterious effects upon you are imminent. Your operation will challenge your body reserves as they have never been tested before. Although under circumstances of ordinary day-to-day living you have been able to avoid the issue of your health, deep down inside you now know that your emotional, dietary, exercise, and personal habits might even determine whether you will survive.

10

Under the Knife

Diseases desperate grown
By desperate appliance are relieved
Or not at all!

                              Hamlet

You enter the glass doorway to the hospital. Crossing the lobby, you pass a doctor in surgical garb talking with a family who sit on the edges of their chairs gazing up apprehensively. In the gift shop, to one side, you see counters with magazines, newspapers, candy, potato chips, and get-well cards. To the rear, a hallway leads to some elevators. You step up to a desk marked *Information* and tell the woman that you are supposed to have surgery the following day. She smiles and says you should report to the admitting office down the hall and to the right. Unsure of where you are going, you walk down the hall and to the right until you find the admitting office. You see another patient signing in for surgery the following day, and you sit in an orange-colored plastic chair to await your turn. When the clerk finishes registering the patient ahead of you, she excuses herself, saying that she has to go admit a patient from the emergency room and will be back in a few minutes.

As you sit there awaiting admission, perhaps you'll begin to feel the reality of your situation. Glancing around the brightly appointed room, you may begin to wonder about the hospital and how well you'll be taken care of there. You may suddenly realize how little you really know about the institution to which you are entrusting your life. What are its qualifications? Is it certified by the Joint Commission of Accreditation of Hospi-

101

tals? Do you know who owns the hospital? Is it a nonprofit community hospital or is it proprietary, run by a profit-making organization? Do you know what facilities are available to you in case you need special care? An intensive care unit? A coronary care unit? Do you know what specialists are available to you? Do you know where you might be transferred in case of complications that cannot be taken care of in your hospital? Do you know if your hospital has the committees and regulations to protect you from incompetent or unscrupulous doctors? Do you know the name of the administrator? The chief of staff?

While you await admission, and the clerk's return, you may realize that you'd feel much more comfortable if you knew the answers to some of those questions. Why didn't you ask more questions about your hospital before you came to be admitted?

If you had, you might have learned, for instance, that most of the approximately seven thousand acute-care hospitals in this country are organized as nonprofit corporations, run by a board of trustees made up of interested and influential members of the communities. Teaching hospitals such as state university hospitals associated with medical schools are also subsidized by education funds and run by representatives of state governments through chancellors and deans of medical schools. Some famous large clinics and some city, county, or federal government hospitals are also nonprofit and are frequently affiliated with university medical schools for teaching. However, approximately two thousand hospitals are proprietary, profit-making institutions owned by doctors and other businessmen and operated for a profit. The boards of trustees are usually comprised of the owner-entrepreneurs to look after their investments.

You might have learned also that the daily affairs of hospitals are controlled by a few different groups. The hospital administrator is appointed by the board of trustees and is supposed to see to the day-to-day running of the department of administrators, personnel, and, of course, budget. The doctors of the hospital control the professional practice through a group of committees which all report to the executive committee, composed of the most influential members of the staff. In most hospitals as many as fifty separate committees meet regularly and make decisions about what happens to patients.

In addition to the credentials committee, the surgical supervisory committee, and the tissue committee, which control the activities of surgeons, there are the records committee, library committee, nurse-physician liaison committee, education and research committee, and innumerable others covering virtually every facet of hospital function.

Is Your Hospital Accredited?

One of the most important facts to know about your hospital is whether it is certified by the Joint Commission of Accreditation of Hospitals. That certification means that the hospital passes periodic inspection aimed at maintaining high standards of patient care. During inspections, the Joint Commission insures that the appropriate committees meet regularly and that the various departments live up to established standards of good practice. In response to patient demands, the Joint Commission has gone so far as to enact a Patient's Bill of Rights, which states that you are entitled:

1) To considerate and respectful care.

2) To obtain from the physician complete current information concerning diagnosis, treatment, and prognosis, in terms you can understand.

3) To obtain from the physician information necessary for informed consent before any procedure or treatment is begun; to information on significant alternatives; and to know the name of the person responsible for the treatment.

4) To refuse treatment to the extent permitted by law and to be informed of the medical consequences of refusal.

5) To every consideration of your privacy concerning your own medical care; persons not directly involved in your care must have your permission to be present at case discussion, consultation, examination, or treatment.

6) To confidentiality of all communications and records pertaining to you.

7) To expect that with its capacity a hospital will make reasonable response to your request for service and not transfer

you to another institution except after you have been given reasons why.

8) To obtain information concerning any relationship of your hospital to other health services so far as your care is concerned, and to existence of any professional relationships among individuals who are treating you.

9) To be advised if the hospital proposes to engage in human experimentation affecting your care and to refuse to participate in such research.

10) To reasonable continuity of care, including postdischarge follow-up.

11) To examine and receive an explanation of your bill no matter who pays it.

12) To know what hospital rules and regulations apply to your conduct as a patient.

Now, that certainly sounds like some important protection for you, doesn't it? Maybe you had better check to see if your hospital is accredited. Look around the admitting office. Do you see it? Perhaps over there on the wall to one side. Yes, there it is, the certificate of the Joint Commission of Accreditation of Hospitals with the little gold seal in one corner. All right, you can settle back now. It's nice to know that you have that going for you. So, just relax.

Is It Dangerous to Your Health?

But perhaps there is another question you should ask yourself. What are you doing here in the first place? Is this hospitalization really necessary? Of course, you say, your doctor wouldn't hospitalize you if it weren't necessary, and the hospital wouldn't let you in if you didn't need to be there. Perhaps. It depends upon your own case and your own hospital, of course, but some experts estimate that nationwide 38 percent of hospitalizations are unnecessary.

It takes money to run hospitals. Hospitals need over 90 percent occupancy just to break even. But because of overbuilding the average hospital in this country only enjoys a 75 percent occupancy rate, and there is a constant excess of one hundred thousand hospital beds nationally. Consequently, in some major cities, hospitals vie with one another for patients, even through advertising and by offering gimmicks like champagne dinners for new parents.

In more than one hospital, campaigns are underway to encourage doctors to admit more patients. Often, not much persuasion is necessary. First of all, patients expect to be hospitalized . . . after all, they have insurance, why not let the nurses and doctors look after them during illness? The doctors, in turn, are reluctant to deny hospitalization for fear the patients and families will think that home treatment is neglectful or malpractice. Besides, it's convenient for the doctors to have their patients in the hospital rather than at home. Surgeons are trained in hospitals and are not accustomed to home management for operations. Yet, as much as 40 percent of surgery now performed in hospitals could be safely accomplished on an "outpatient" basis at a cost of one-fourth to one-half of in-hospital care.

Some enlightened communities have developed out-patient Surgicenters where patients come in for only a few hours for their operations then return home for recuperation—so-called come-and-go surgery. D & C, hernia operations, urinary bladder examinations, and most hermorrhoid, breast, varicose vein, eye, and plastic surgery can be done safely without expensive hospitalization. Patients can recuperate at home with loved ones and family instead of in a hospital.

You say you would prefer to be in the hospital with nurses and aides to take care of your comforts and maybe flowers in your room? Why not? Why shouldn't you be in the protective arms of medical professionals? Well, it turns out that, like most aspects of medical care, hospitalization is not without hazards. In fact, despite lofty goals of caring for patients and saving lives, hospitals are extremely dangerous places.

The accident rates in some hospitals are higher than in most other industries. Seven percent of patients suffer significant injuries while in hospitals. One in every fifty children in American hospitals experiences a serious accident. Indeed, accident records are so high that some hospitals could be closed by the Department of Health.

Accidents are probably inevitable in hospitals where so many sick people cannot safely care for themselves and where dangerous diagnostic tests and therapeutic regimens are performed every day. Patients fall out of bed, fracturing bones. Intravenous fluids are allowed to run too fast, drowning patients. Others are permitted to run dry, threatening to kill patients with air bubbles. Infants are dropped to the floor, patients are given the wrong medicines, bowels are perforated with thermometers or enema tubes, and needles and plastic catheters are lost inside patients' bodies.

Patients have been fed soap solutions instead of antacids. One man drank his own urine instead of fruit juice. At least one woman suffered an explosion inside her vagina when a cautery instrument ignited ether, which had mistakenly been used instead of alcohol for disinfectant. In one hospital, a patient who had suffered a stroke died after being deserted on an elevator for twelve hours without food or water.

In at least two hospitals, pipes carrying anesthetic gases were mixed up so that patients were killed by nitrous oxide instead of receiving the precious oxygen they needed. In another case, an oxygen tube was mistakenly connected to a gastric suction device so that volumes of gas were forced into the patient's stomach until it ruptured. In another foul-up, a patient was actually given cement to drink instead of the liquid barium for special X rays. Inside, the concrete formed a perfect cast of the stomach and upper intestine.

As impossible as it may seem, another patient was given cyanide instead of a glucose solution for a diabetes test. An anesthesiologist fatally injected ether instead of a barbiturate into a patient's bloodstream.

Every technological innovation of modern scientific medicine brings with it new, sometimes lethal, accident potentials. Respirators go haywire, pumps break, and pacemakers fail. Indeed, in one intensive care unit, the wires from electronic devices were crossed or short-circuited and patients were actually electrocuted in their own beds.

In the scientific milieu of modern hospital care, however, accidents are not the only risk. In some university hospitals, for instance, twenty percent of patients suffer a complication actually caused by their medical care. Half of those are complications of drugs—mistakes in therapy, side reactions, and allergies. Furthermore, hospital-acquired infections are an increasing threat, accounting for as many as one hundred thousand deaths a year.

But not only are hospitals dangerous to your health, they also might not be as comfortable as you anticipate. Through interviews and questionnaires, the administrators of one hospital learned that 17 percent of patients said they would be unwilling to return for additional care. Many found the rooms noisy, the food inedible, and information impossible to obtain. In most hospitals, patients are expected to live by rules and regulations, and by the daily routine of doctors and nurses. All too often, patients are kept waiting sometimes for hours because of inefficient laboratory and X-ray facilities, which cater more to the financial remuneration of doctors than to the medical needs of patients. Reports of patients left alone for hours in wheelchairs, crying for help and calling for nurses, are not always exaggerations, and the old story about patients being awakened from a sound sleep to be administered sleeping pills is all too often true.

How can it be that hospitals, which are supposed to be lifesaving institutions, can be responsible for harming, even causing deaths of patients? How can it be that so many children admitted to hospitals suffer injuries? How can it be that patients are sometimes neglected, that the Patients' Bill of Rights is not more strictly enforced? How can hospitals be so inefficient if they are accredited by the Joint Commission and are run by professional administrators and doctors?

Commissions and Committees

A closer look at the activities of the Joint Commission may at least partially explain some of the dilemma. To start with, 25 percent of American hospitals are not even accredited, so are not inspected at all. Additionally, each year some hospitals are placed on probation because of discrepancies, but allowed to continue operating on probation until the next inspection.

Even certification does not guarantee that hospitals are up to standard. After all, the hospitals are inspected only every three years. Even at that rate, the Joint Commission is badly under-staffed. Each inspection is required to evaluate eleven hospitals per month, a rate which is wholly inadequate for an in-depth review of the hospital records and functions. Besides, the Joint Commission does not directly regulate hospitals. Its stated role is to advise and help, not to criticize. For instance, the inspection teams might be concerned about whether or not the committees meet regularly, but do not have time to evaluate what the committees decided during those meetings. Aware of the relative superficiality of the inspection, most hospital staffs begin hurriedly correcting known deficiencies a few weeks before the inspectors arrive. Medical records librarians scurry about getting doctors to complete and sign records, secretaries labor over minutes of meetings, and medical charts are reviewed for completeness. It happens in almost every hospital just before every inspection. Afterward, the staff breathes a sigh of relief and settles back into their usual something-less-than-optimal performance. Because of these tactics, Department of Health, Education, and Welfare spot checks of 105 *accredited* hospitals showed significant health and safety deficiencies, including failure to meet fire regulations, inadequate patient records, improper drug records, and below-standard food services.

Hospital administrators have a lot to say about the budgets and business practices of hospitals, but they can hardly be held responsible for the practice standards of medical care. In most hospitals, administrators simply act as advocates of what the powerful physician-dominated committees decide.

Hospital committees are also frequently inefficient, unable to resolve the problems put before them. Doctors become involved, for instance, in personnel problems, nursing programs, and administrative matters for which their opinions are invalid and might be better left to experts in those particular areas. Furthermore, bickering among doctors on the committees is commonplace, and the whole system is controlled by the small cadre of the most influential members of the staff who sit on the executive committee and who frequently predetermine in private meetings what a particular decision will be. Consequently, nowhere else is it more appropriate to apply the adage that a camel is a horse designed by a committee.

Remember all those accidents we talked about? Yes, they are the responsibility of the Safety Committee. In one hospital, the Disaster Committee, a body made up of doctors and nurses and administrators, was charged with formulating and implementing a plan to be used for the care of victims of a catastrophe. After a full year of discussions a master plan was completed. Only a few months later came a real disaster—rioting in the city streets. Under the conditions of a real-life situation, the carefully prepared Disaster Plan was scrapped within minutes when it became obvious that it was useless for the situation. The nurses and doctors on duty simply responded reasonably to the needs as they presented themselves.

Hospital committees can also become bureaucratic, at times almost paralyzing progress. In one hospital, for instance, the respiratory therapists devised a little form that they could conveniently use in their work. They were advised that their form would have to be approved by the Special Care Committee, which oversaw, among other things, the respiratory care unit. After discussion at two committee meetings, the members approved the form. But not so fast, said one member. First, the form had to be approved by, yes, the Forms Committee. Six months later, the respiratory therapy technicians were still using scratch paper.

In many hospitals the inefficiency is made worse because the committees are sometimes used as power bases by ambitious doctors. In many hospitals, certain chairmen of departments are well known to be hardheaded fellows who stubbornly refuse to allow anything to pass the committee unless it suits them personally. In one hospital, a powerful department head used the Research and Education Committee to besmirch and blackball those individuals whom he considered undesirable.

You can hope that this sort of thing doesn't go on inside your hospital, that your hospital is run smoothly and in the best interests of patients. But as you sit in the admitting office waiting to sign into the hospital, you might just begin to wonder how your hospital would be rated and what you can do to protect yourself.

Signing In

. . . Oh, here comes the admitting clerk. She's finished with the patient in the emergency room and is ready to sign you in. Try not to be irritated about the delay. After all, your registration is being looked after by the Admissions Committee, and surveys show that only about half of patients admitted to hospitals get from the door up to their rooms in less than an hour.

After you complete a few forms and show your insurance papers or make a substantial cash deposit, you will be directed to sign a legal document. Read it. The form is required because the doctors, nurses, or other personnel cannot treat you without your permission—to do so would constitute assault and battery. So, to protect the hospital, you are required to give permission in writing.

Remember, that form was made up by the administrators and lawyers to protect the interests of the hospital, and you may find that they've slipped in a few phrases in small print that are not necessarily in *your* best interest. You'll have to sign to get your medical care, but at least read the forms so you know what you're signing.

You might find, for instance, that you are allowing the doctors to perform additional care about which you have not been informed. You might find, also that you are signing an agreement to pay 18 percent annual interest and to pay costs of a bill collector if you are unable to pay your hospital bill on time. You may also be permitting the hospital to disclose all information about your hospital record to agents under contract with the hospital, insurance companies, and your employer. You will learn that the hospital is not responsible for your valuables.

Most importantly, you may be agreeing not to hold anyone liable for harm that might come to you through routine care— things like accidents. In addition, you might be asked to sign an operative permit. In it, you acknowledge that you have had the

out about what's going on and what's going to happen.

There might have been a complete program about the hospital and about your own particular operation on closed-circuit television in your room except for one thing. After the proposal was initiated in the Patient Care Committee by a nurse, then passed by the Communications Committee, Nursing Committee, Public Relations Committee, Equipment Committee, Special Appropriations Committee, and Budget Committee, it was turned down by the Executive Committee. Two of the older doctors vehemently disagreed with the proposal and convinced the other members to cancel the plan because, they said, patients don't want all that information, it was too expensive, the money could be used for redecorating the doctors' lounge, and that it might make doctors liable legally if they didn't comply with what was shown on the television. So, you'll have to wait until your doctor comes for information.

Hospital Routine

While you wait, however, you may have plenty to occupy your time. During the next few hours, many things are liable to happen. You may have blood taken from your arm vein, for instance. Your temperature may be taken again. You may go to the radiology department for X rays. Someone may come into your room with a razor and shave part of your body. You may be administered special tests, an electrocardiogram, breathing exercises. You may be measured, elevated on platforms, tilted on movable tables, be given intravenous injections of diagnostic dyes or isotope solutions, wheeled down hallways and in and out of elevators on stretchers or wheelchairs, poked and rubbed with cold instruments and solutions, and given any number of potions to swallow. This is a time to be careful.

During these day-to-day, routine activities accidents can happen. Remember, hospitals are potentially dangerous. If you want to protect yourself, you'll have to be careful. When a nurse starts to take you to X ray, for instance, you might just ask what the test is for and why you are having it. If a medication is brought to you, by all means ask what it is and what it is for.

You might take a lesson from some of the "professional" patients who can be found in many Veteran Administration or Public Health Service hospitals. Because of disabilities from injuries or chronic illnesses, these patients have been forced to spend years of their lives in hospitals. Consequently, they are "ward wise" and have learned to protect themselves. They have been in medical facilities enough to have witnessed or have had inflicted upon themselves the results of human errors of hospital practice.

If you ever had the opportunity to observe these savvy patients, you would notice that they check every detail of their own care. They move about the hospital ward with the wariness of a fox who has just heard the cry of tally-ho. They won't accept a pill with which they are unfamiliar, and they can be seen reminding a nurse when it's time for an important treatment or medication. By asking questions about everything, they know what should and should not be done. They help other patients, too.

In any VA hospital ward, a doctor looking for a patient might quite likely be advised by one of these ward-wise fellows that the patient has gone to X ray for a gallbladder test, for instance. These ward-wise patients can sometimes actually prevent mistakes. Some of them would make excellent members of Safety Committees.

You will probably never find it necessary to gain the insight of these professional patients. But you can ask questions. Remember, for the nurses your medications and treatments are routine, but you only have one patient to be concerned about—yourself. So, if someone approaches you trying to insert some device into your nose or ear—or any other bodily orifice for that matter—ask about it. You might discover that it isn't supposed to be for you, and you may want to tell the nurse to stick it somewhere else.

Sometime during the afternoon or evening, your doctor will come to see you. In teaching hospitals, three or four interns or residents may also examine you. If you chose your surgeon carefully or if the house doctors are helpful, you may have your questions answered and your anxieties allayed. If not, your nagging unanswered questions may begin to raise doubts and fears.

Prepare a written list ahead of time, if necessary, but for your own good, don't go to the operating room unless your questions have all been answered and your fears resolved.

The anesthesiologist should stop in to see you, too. This is the visit during which you're supposed to find out about your anesthetic and state your preferences. It is also the time to get to know the anesthesiologist who is going to take your life into his hands the next morning.

Sometime during the early evening you will be served supper. If your hospital is an exception, the meal may be attractive, nutritious, and palatable. But in many hospitals, food is over-cooked and stored in steam tables so that by the time it is served it is unappetizing and flavorless. Furthermore, it may not be nutritious.

Surveys done by a reputable university report that nutrition does not receive enough attention in hospitals. Diets are often inadequate even to maintain health. Even patients with known protein abnormalities were sometimes not fed therapeutic diets. Furthermore, withholding of meals for laboratory and X-ray studies, failure to measure food intake, and prolonged use of intravenous fluids add to the inadequate nutrition found in some hospitals.

If you are not able to ingest adequate calories and essential foodstuffs in the hospital to help you through surgery, you will be doubly glad that you prepared for your operation at home with a high protein diet and adequate vitamins and minerals.

In the evening you will be put to bed, and usually offered some tranquilizers or sleeping pills. Perhaps you would prefer your meditation or yoga to relax you, thereby avoiding the potential side effects and complications of drugs. It's a good time for your self-relaxing techniques to lower your anxieties so that you can sleep soundly. If the patient sharing your room doesn't fall out of bed, or if a critically ill patient isn't brought in during the night, you may sleep soundly. You may be awakened by a nurse giving you some preoperative medication by injection. If you've talked with your doctors ahead of time, you will receive only those drugs that are necessary. Then you will be put flat on your back on a stretcher and will begin to see the world from a new, and perhaps disconcerting, perspective, watching the ceiling pass by above you as you are wheeled down corridors, through elevators, and into surgery.

In the operating room, the shiny equipment and bright lights may stun you at first. It may be cold, too. The temperature is set for the heavy gowns and drapes used during surgery. But your preoperative medications may have taken effect and you feel relaxed, even giddy. The anesthetic machine is ready and the doctor talks calmly, preparing you for anesthesia.

As you slide onto the operating table, a safety strap is fastened across your upper thighs to prevent you from falling off onto the floor. Your surgeon may step into the room and tell you not to worry. An intravenous line will be put into your arm and the anesthesiologist may give you some oxygen by mask. If you are to have spinal anesthesia, you will be rolled onto one side and an injection made into your back, then you'll be given sedatives to help you sleep. If you're having a general anesthetic, some medication will be injected through the intravenous tubing.

Briefly clinging to cognition, you glance furtively around the room once more. You see the bright overhead light. You see the shining steel instruments on the table nearby. You are aware of the masked faces of the doctors and nurses looking down at you. Suddenly, reality fades. You hear bells or see colors or your mind flashes upon some almost forgotten memories as you slip through the twilight zone. Then, with a sensation of being swept rapidly backward, you fall into the abyss of unconsciousness.

11
Ouch!

———————— • ————————

Pleasure is oft a visitant;
But pain clings cruelly to us.
                        Keats

In the recovery room after your operation, as you slowly awaken from the anesthetic, and regain consciousness, your attention will be constrained to one urgent and exquisite sensation —pain. Why didn't anyone say how much it was going to hurt? Perhaps it's because people don't like to talk about pain. It's too unpleasant. Not only that, nature seems to have provided a saving grace—most people forget about pain they have suffered as though a state of amnesia protects them from the unbearable.

Pain is probably the primary biological model of all human suffering, and it is meticulously avoided by all except masochists or religious fanatics. Even if your doctor carefully informed you about your surgery, he may have neglected to mention pain. Friends and relatives may have told you about their operations in great detail, but they probably left out one important facet—pain. Yet, whatever operation you have, it will hurt postoperatively.

You may be given medications—many medications—but it will still hurt. It will hurt when you move. It will hurt when you breathe deeply. It will hurt even more when you cough, sneeze, or vomit. Nothing can make you feel so helpless as pain; it seems to take over your whole body and force you into passive submission. Yet, there is much you can do to help yourself when the pain of surgery strikes. In fact, just knowing more about pain can help you. Your knowledge about pain and your mental

116

and emotional attitude toward it can do more to help you through your postoperative period than anything else. Furthermore, you can learn to control your pain with a few simple techniques, which can work better than even the most powerful drugs.

Let's start by emphasizing that pain is not a disease. No one ever died of pain. Pain is a symptom. When injuries, tumors, swellings, inflammation, or poor circulation wreak their effects upon living tissues, nerve endings are stimulated and pain is the result. But pain is not a single experience. Rather, it is the result of complex interactions of many external stimuli and inner feelings.

To start with, at least two kinds of pain impulses arise in our bodies. They travel different pathways to the brain to produce a variety of sensations, all of them very unpleasant. To experience the differences in the two types of pain you need only slap the top of one hand with the fingers of the other. If you observe carefully, you will recognize two separate sensations. The first is an immediate, sharp pain occuring exactly where your fingers struck your hand. The second is a slower, duller, and more diffuse, seeming to gather sensation from a broader area. The first type of pain is characteristic of injuries like bullet and knife wounds or burns. It is more prominent in the superficial areas of the body just under the skin. The second, slower type of pain is found deeper in the body and is more characteristic of chronic pain from tumors or headaches. After an operation, you will experience both types of pain, the sharp pain of your skin incision and the aching pain from deep within your body.

Though they are transmitted at different velocities, both types of pain travel through the bodily network of nerves, which connect like the twigs of the branches and the branches to the trunk of a tree, finally forming the spinal cord. The nerve fibers then pass up the spinal cord where they connect like wires into a switchboard in an area at the base of the brain called the arousal center. From there they are sorted out to particular regions of the brain, each with certain functions for the appreciation of and the reaction to the stimulus.

Some fibers transmit the painful sensation to the sensory area of the brain so that you can tell where the pain is located, how intense it is, and what kind of stimulus caused it. Other pain fibers travel from the arousal area to the medulla, the center that controls basic bodily functions. There they trigger responses that result in visceral manifestations such as salivation, pupil dilatation, vomiting, sweating, rapid heartbeat, or even involuntary urination and defecation.

Still other fibers connect from the arousal area to the so-called higher brain centers, those mysterious areas of gray matter in which awareness, reasoning, and emotions arise. The effect of these painful stimuli upon the higher brain centers produces a complex, overwhelming experience known as suffering. If these connecting fibers are cut, as is done in prefontal lobotomy, for instance, the patient can still feel, locate, and identify painful stimuli, but does not suffer and, in fact, often feels nonchalant or euphoric.

Pain Can Be Modified

Because of the variability and complexity of activity in the so-called higher brain centers, pain can be remarkably modified by the awareness and emotions generated in those centers. For instance, not only do different people experience pain to varying degrees, but the same individual will react differently, depending upon the activity in the higher centers. Selective perception, fatigue, mood, and anxiety all alter one's ability to tolerate pain. Furthermore, it is through these higher centers that you can effectively control your own feelings of pain and your reactions to it.

Selective perception is the way our minds choose which of the thousands of stimuli to think about or to perceive. As an illustration, if you pause a moment to pay attention to your shoes on your feet or your clothing around your shoulders, you will be able to sense the feelings of pressure and rubbing of the fabrics against your skin. Now, those nerve impulses were constantly being passed from your skin to your brain, but you didn't appreciate them until you chose to focus upon them. That's selective perception.

Because of this phenomenon, people can focus upon pain to make it worse. Some individuals have actually been overcome by painful stimuli that under ordinary circumstances might go almost unnoticed. During medical school, for instance, many students experience painful symptoms associated with the diseases they are currently studying. They are actually feeling normal gas bubbles and movements of their muscles or intestines because their focus of attention has been drawn to their own bodies.

Motivation also plays a role. For instance, a bump on the knee might necessitate X rays, medications, and bed rest if it occured at work but go almost unnoticed on a ski slope. Many symptoms of psychosomatic disease are only exaggerations and selective perception of normal bodily feelings.

By heightening activity in the higher brain centers, fatigue, anxiety, and fear play an important role in the experience of pain. When one is tired or worried, painful stimuli seem much more exquisite. These interactions can lead to a vicious cycle, pain causing suffering . . . which increases anxiety . . . which then heightens the pain . . . causing more suffering . . . which increases anxiety, etcetera.

But the elements in the higher brain centers can work in your favor, also. You can actually block and modify painful stimuli. Hypnosis, for instance, may eliminate pain by blocking impulses from the arousal center to the higher centers. But selective perception can be effective, too. Soldiers wounded in battle have sometimes fought on for hours, unaware of bullet or shrapnel wounds because their minds had selected sheer survival as the exclusive focus of attention.

Furthermore, decreasing your fear and anxiety—factors so important in your preparation for surgery—can change a vicious cycle into a beneficial cycle, lowered anxiety giving decreased pain . . . which relieves suffering . . . which then lowers anxiety . . . giving decreased pain . . . which relieves suffering, etcetera. Indeed, these factors of the pain experience have been shown to be more powerful than the strongest drugs, and are the tools with which you can most effectively help yourself after an operation.

One reason why you can control your own pain by mental

and emotional techniques is that your own body can produce painkilling substances that are even more powerful than narcotics. Recent studies have demonstrated that under the proper conditions of meditation, biofeedback, and hypnosis, the human brain actually produces a substance called *endorphan,* which has all the painkilling properties of narcotics but none of the dangerous side effects. Just think, with the proper attitude, selective perception, and lowered anxiety, you can provide yourself with relief of pain without any of the side effects of drugs.

Pain Clings

Another important factor to understand about pain is its tendency to "cling cruelly to us." Paradoxically, as romantic poets have long observed, life's pleasures are often fleeting, while pain seems only to get worse. This phenomenon has roots in basic neurological function. Pleasurable sensations always decrease with continued stimulation. For instance, the second piece of apple pie never tastes quite so good as the first, and a third or fourth helping can become downright nauseating. If constantly repeated, even the pleasant feeling of a gentle stroking of the skin will gradually become irritating, then extremely unpleasant. The nerves become "satiated" and their ability to transmit pleasant sensations ceases—even reverses.

Painful nerves, on the other hand, when repeatedly stimulated, tend to become more and more sensitive, actually heightening the sensation and increasing the pain. The repeated painful sticking of the skin with a hypodermic needle will grow more and more excruciating until it is finally unbearable. The sensations along the nerve fibers seem actually to increase instead of becoming satiated. The effect may be due in part to increased anxiety associated with pain, but mostly it is the normal physiological response of the nerves themselves. This phenomenon can be observed on a chronic basis in those individuals who have undergone multiple operations and can no longer tolerate even the slight pain of a needle.

Thus, the unremitting pain of surgery, if left unchecked, can gradually become unbearable. The suffering it causes can literally make you want to lie down and die. It can make you reluctant to move, unable to breathe deeply, cough, or exercise, thereby inhibiting all those activities necessary to prevent complications. Obviously, the pain of surgery must be relieved or you may not survive your operation.

Painkillers

When most people consider relief of pain their thoughts may well turn to television commercials about sinus congestion, neuritis, neuralgia, backache, or arthritis. They may think about all those medications, some with added ingredients, each of which has supposedly been proved by doctors to be more effective than all the others. Most doctors also think of drugs as the way to relieve pain. Drugs are quick and easy to use and do not require the effort and time of other methods of pain control involving the higher brain centers. Not only that, doctors are the recipients of the same mass advertising as is bestowed upon the general public through television commercials.

The variety of painkilling drugs available for doctors to prescribe is innumerable. Each one is claimed to be better than all the others. To prove their untenable claims, drug companies engage in continual marketing campaigns. It starts in medical school when the students are given little black bags and stethoscopes and free trips by the drug companies.

For practicing physicians, over fifteen thousand drug salesmen and representative nationwide visit medical offices and hospitals regularly, leaving samples and gifts such as calendars, ballpoint pens, and other office supplies. Doctors' mailboxes are filled daily with advertisements from drug compainies. One doctor measured his mail and found that he received thirty-five pounds of drug company advertising material in one month. In all, drug companies spend over a billion dollars a year promoting their products to doctors. In the name of free enterprise, these ordinary business activities can be justified. But doctors, who are supposed to be scientists and dedicated practitioners, succumb to the advertising—and that cannot be justified.

The first line of medical treatment taken by physicians is usually some kind of drug. In hospital wards, patient after patient can be found receiving eight or ten different drugs for everything from headache to hangnails. Nurses shake their heads in despair as they pass out the drugs the doctors have ordered. To some observers, the overuse of drugs in hospitals is even more disgraceful than the dope scene on our city streets.

Why *not* use these lifesaving, healing medicines? Why shouldn't patients have the benefit of therapeutic chemicals developed through years of research especially antibiotics, which alone have saved millions of lives? Why? Because surveys have shown that only about half the antibiotics prescribed in hospitals are justified. Even that might not be so bad were it not for the fact that antibiotics can kill. Thousands have died from penicillin alone.

The record of painkillers is even worse. The benefits from their extended and massive use may not have been worth the side effects and deaths they cause. First of all, whether these drugs are really effective is open to serious question. The claims made by the drug companies in the doctors' advertising are no more scientifically valid than those you see on television.

The research data gathered by the drug companies is often not statistically significant. In fact, one survey showed that only 5 percent of clinical trials of drugs were scientifically valid. The Drug Efficacy Study Groups of the FDA found that twenty-three hundred claims of therapeutic benefits of drugs were without any evidence whatsoever. Only two of every five drugs were judged to be clearly effective. Many of the totally inneffective drugs have been taken off the market, and a large number of "possibly" effective ones are under investigation. How can it be that drug companies can make so many unfounded claims?

Most clinical tests of drugs are accomplished by doctors in their own practices who are paid by the companies to use them, a totally inadequate method for conducting a scientific study. Appallingly, one doctor was discovered to have submitted the exact test results for a dozen or more different drugs, collecting his fee for each test. But even when doctors are trying to be honest about their studies, they cannot conduct a valid study simply by asking patients if they feel better. It's just not statistically valid unless strict controls using placebos and "double-blind" techniques are built into the studies.

But even careful scientific research of pain relief is virtually impossible. That's because of those higher brain centers, which modify pain so remarkably. A research subject in a laboratory just does not react in the same way to pain as a patient experiencing the anxiety and fears associated with disease, hospitatilization, and surgery.

More importantly, independent research conducted at some university centers indicates that only one third of postoperative patients experience relief of their pain with narcotics. What's more, another third respond as well to sterile water as they do to the drugs. That means that fewer than half the patients receiving pain medications postoperatively derive any benefit whatsoever from the drugs. Add to that the patients who would respond satisfactorily to safer methods of pain control, such as hypnosis, acupuncture, meditation, or breathing techniques, and, at the very least, one must conclude that the use of drugs for pain postoperatively could be drastically reduced.

Still, why not use them if many patients do obtain relief? Certainly, postoperative patients cannot be left in severe pain. Because even if the pain-relieving drugs were effective, there are still valid reasons to reconsider their extensive use, most importantly, that all these drugs have significant side effects and risks.

Although no one has died from pain per se, many people have died from the drugs used to relieve pain. In some hospitals, one in every ten patients suffers complications of drugs—mistakes in therapy, side reactions, and allergies. Furthermore, evidence indicates that addiction to some drugs is caused more by doctors than by illicit drug traffic. The fact that so many doctors themselves become addicted is testimony enough to the lack of restraint in the use of drugs.

How dangerous are pain-relieving drugs? To get an idea, you might be interested in some information available to docotrs but not usually obtained by patients. For instance, the most frequently prescribed injectable pain medication has two benefits, sedation and pain relief. In the drug literature available to doctors, a description of these desirable effects requires about two inches on a printed column. In contrast, the accompanying undesirable, even dangerous side reactions to the drug requires a column twenty-four inches long! There are twenty-five warnings, eleven precautions, thirty-seven adverse reactions, and seventeen symptoms of overdosage. Disconcertingly, these untoward reactions include pain at the injection site, local tissue irritation, itching, skin rashes, lightheadedness, weakness, dizziness, headache, sedation, agitation, nausea, vomiting, tremor, sweating, uncoordinated muscle movements, hallucinations, visual disturbances, disorientation, dry mouth, biliary tract spasm, constipation, flushing, rapid heart rate, slow heart rate, palpitations, fainting, urinary retention, respiratory depression, circulatory depression, respiratory arrest, cardiac arrest, and death. More importantly, these reactions are not only printed in books. They are a part of routine postoperative care in every hospital, and doctors and nurses see them all the time.

Perhaps you're beginning to feel confused. Postoperative pain interferes with your ability to do those things that help you recover, and pain medications can be harmful because of their serious side effects. What are you to do? Will you have to suffer through, hoping for the best? Not at all.

No one would suggest that most people can get through operations without some medications. After all, these drugs are extremely helpful if used correctly. But all too often they are prescribed unnecessarily, when relief of anxiety or supportive counseling might be more effective. Postoperatively, patients frequently ask for medications because of fear of pain rather than from an actual feeling of discomfort. But knowing about the risks might encourage you to keep the use of drugs to a minimum. Perhaps when that little ache begins you'll think twice before asking for pain medication unless the pain becomes much worse. Perhaps when the nurse drops by to give you a routine pain shot, you'll refuse, recognizing that if you don't absolutely need the medication, you're better off avoiding possible side effects. With the proper attitude and decreased anxiety, many patients can go through major operations using aspirin alone.

Perhaps you could be one of those patients who can undergo surgery with minimal use of drugs, avoiding narcotics altogether. You already know about relief of anxiety and fears through increasing your knowledge and information about your operation. You know about various methods of meditation and yoga, which can improve your ability to withstand an operation.

The LaMaze breathing techniques have transformed childbirth from painful torture into a pleasant, fulfilling experience for many women. These breathing techniques have not been adopted by anesthesiologists or surgeons, but nurses and patients have discovered excellent results using them for postoperative pain. Furthermore, meditation, hypnosis, and acupuncture, which we discussed as methods of anesthesia, are especially useful postoperatively. You may want to consider using some of these techniques instead of drugs for control of your pain. If so, discuss them with your doctors and anesthesiologists ahead of time. They may be more available than you think, and they may be just what you need to avoid drugs. Whatever you decide, just knowing about the nature of pain and its relief will help you through your operation more comfortably and safely.

12
Getting Better

*Healing is a matter of time, but it is sometimes
also a matter of opportunity.*
Hippocrates

Now all your careful preparations will pay off. You found
out all about your illness and operation, came to a personal
decision, and are confident you are receiving the best possible
treatment. You prepared yourself psychologically and physically to withstand the stress of surgery. You chose your surgeon
and anesthesiologist carefully so that by their superb skills
you've come through the operation. You're on the road to recovery. You've learned about potential complications and have
resolved to do whatever you can to prevent them in your own
case. You've survived the worst of it, and if you can just keep up
the good work, you'll be well soon.

You now have the opportunity to help yourself get better. If
you choose, you can just lie there, passively allowing your
doctors and nurses to take care of you. If you have accepted or
requested high doses of potent drugs, you may remain in a daze
for another day or so, and if you have only put minimal effort
into ambulation, deep breathing, and coughing, you have not
adequately protected yourself against respiratory and circulatory complications. In either case, you will have delayed your
recovery and subjected yourself to increased risks.

If, however, you decided to take charge of your own recovery,
accepting only minimal medications and actively participating
in your postoperative program, you can help prevent complications and insure your return to good health. You will find that

126

you are quite alert, and feel better than you had thought you would. Sure, there's that bothersome pain at the operative incision, but your selective perception, positive attitude, calmness, breathing exercises or meditation can help that. There are those annoying tubes in your nose, IVs in your arm, that packing, casts, drains, bandages, or whatever packaging might be appropriate to your particular case. But you are doing all right, can breathe deeply if you want to, and can move around in bed easily. So, why just lie there? Why not get out of bed?

Aside from needing some help because you are a little unsure of your equilibrium and all the medical paraphernalia, there is no reason why you shouldn't get out of bed. Your nurses know that the best thing for you is to get up, so they'll most likely be along soon to help you. But when nurses get too busy with medication, schedules, treatments, and charting, the first item to be neglected usually is patient ambulation. So, if the nurse doesn't come to help you soon, complain and insist upon some exercise. Soon you'll be up on your feet and ready to help yourself get better.

The Four W's

To help prevent complications you will need to learn about the basic principles of postoperative care. Whereas in grammar school you learned the *three R's*, you now must think of the *four Ws* — wind, water, walking, and wound.

Wind is for breathing. You may have noticed that after your operation the first thing doctors or nurses do when examining you is to put a stethoscope on your chest and listen to your breathing. They're checking for signs of decreased lung expansion and pneumonia. They know that the lungs are the most common site of complications and one of the most frequent causes of death postoperatively. They know that surgery stresses the lungs in many ways, predisposing to complications.

As you lie on an operating table, or later in bed, your chest is compressed and your diaphragm's movements limited so that the little air sacs in the most peripheral portions of your lungs collapse. If left unopened, the result is atelectasis, then pneumonia. Your doctor may prescribe suction of your airway with catheters or breathing treatments with respirators, but the very best way of all for opening up and cleaning out your lungs is by your own efforts. You will have to breathe deeply even though it may hurt your incision. You will have to cough and bring up the phlegm that tends to collect in the bronchial tubes. It's all a little difficult at first but with help you can do it.

As soon as you learn how, you can take care of your lungs yourself. The nurses have time to help you two or three times a day. On your own you can deep-breathe and cough every hour if you want to. If you do that, you'll actually prevent those dread pulmonary postopertive complications. Again, the fewer drugs you take the better. And aren't you glad you started exercising before you came into the hospital?

Water is needed for your bodily fluid balance and kidney function. Those intravenous fluids you have been receiving are to prevent dehydration because you have been unable to eat or drink before and after your operation and because you lost some blood by bleeding and fluid by evaporation during your operation. Without intravenous fluids you would become dehydrated and your kidneys would no longer function.

During the operative phase, you'll have to rely upon your surgeons to supervise your fluid replacement and the nurses to administer it properly. But some of those ward-wise patients do ask about intravenous fluids and keep an eye on them, letting the nurses know if the fluids are infusing too slowly or too rapidly—or if the bottle runs dry, allowing air into the veins.

Once you begin eating, however, there is a lot you can do to help your fluid balance. Be sure to drink enough liquids and don't leave food behind. Observe for yourself that you are urinating the usual amount, not often enough or too often, and notify your nurses if you have pain or burning.

Walking is necessary to avoid inflammation and blood clots in your legs. This may be the most important of all your postoperative efforts. Ambulation increases the circulation in your legs 50 percent and will help prevent those dread clots that can go to the lungs and cause sudden death. But it's even more important than that. An upright posture is much better for your lung function, allowing the diaphragm to move freely and the chest muscles to elevate the ribs for deep breathing.

You will probably be asked to walk once or twice a day, but the way you do it is important. Some patients hang onto the nurse and beg to get back into bed. Don't do that. A strong aggressive approach, walking as erect and as far as you can, will help you immensely. By the way, your ability to control your pain will greatly enhance your ability to ambulate.

Wound care is obviously important. Not only must the incision heal properly, but infection must be avoided. The most important factors in healing and antisepsis of wounds are accomplished by your nutritional preparation and then by your surgeon in the operating room. His careful technique and attention to detail will determine how well your incision heals.

For you, it is important to observe the wound carefully and to report any changes to your doctor. If, for instance, you realize that your incision was hurting less every day and then began to hurt more, tell your surgeon. It could be the first sign of infection. Also, if you detect a pulling or a popping sensation, tell your doctor. It could be that you've pulled a stitch.

As your incision improves, it will become more and more comfortable and will gradually grow even stronger than the surrounding normal tissue. The scar will stay pink for a few months, then will gradually become the color of your skin as the protein connective tissue matures.

Of course, depending upon your operation, there may be many specific aspects of recovery—casts, traction, supports, bindings, tubes, drains, soaks, irrigations, catheters, or monitors. You may want to ask about these forms of treatment, but the management of them will, of course, rest with your doctors and nurses. For you, however, the *four Ws* will suffice to help you. If you remember wind, water, walking, and wound, and apply your preventive measures energetically, you will help yourself immeasurably.

Pay attention to how you feel. Up to now the important thing has been for you to ask questions. This is the time for you to give answers, and the best and earliest diagnostic signs are how you feel. So, tell your nurses and doctors anything that seems significant. If you notice a fever or chill, let the nurse know. If you note a change in the color of the phlegm from your throat, tell someone. I can't enumerate all the things to watch for, but just be aware that any change is significant, and never hesitate to talk to someone about it.

Take Responsibility for Yourself

Each day you will be able to assume more responsibility for yourself. Remember, although you can't control all the medical technicalities, you can still assume the responsibility for what drugs you take and how vigorously you want to exercise .

As tubes and intravenous lines are removed, you can begin to eat, and you'll find even more freedom. You can pay attention to your diet, for instance. You know you have been losing protein—lots of protein—and those intravenous bottles only contained sugar. You know you need protein to heal your wound. Look at what you were brought from the kitchen. Does it have enough protein? Bread, potatoes, cold cereals, and fruit juices do not have very much protein.

Ask your doctor about your diet. Ask the nurses about your diet. If your hospital food is not adequate, does not contain the necessary protein, vitamins, and minerals, ask to talk to the hospital dietician personally. Some patients have even asked family or friends to bring in food. A bowl of chicken soup might be a good start, but even more extensive supplements have been provided to some patients by concerned relatives.

The next question is when to go home. Most patients stay in the hospital too long after surgery. The same factors that influence doctors to hospitalize patients unnecessarily also come to bear upon length of stay. Many doctors are concerned about legal liabilities, that if things don't go well, patients and their families—or even a jury—might consider early discharge from the hospital negligent. Other doctors are just too conservative. They want to keep their operative procedures under their control For instance, most surgeons keep patients in the hospital after hemorrhoidectomy until after a bowel movement. But there is no reason why well-informed patients could not go home on the day of the operation if they are aware of the problem of bowel movements after hemorrhoidectomy. One surgeon nature of the operation and treatment fully explained to you. That's the part where you're supposed to be told about all the substantive risks, alternatives, and complications.

Maybe there is some wording or ideas in the permits you don't exactly agree with or that at least need some clarification. But it's too late to quibble now, isn't it? I mean, you've got to have the operation, and you've prepared yourself medically. It seems a little unfair. This isn't any time to be making a legal decision . . . Well, let me tell you about a young lawyer friend.

He was away from home on business in a strange town and was suddenly struck with severe pain from kidney stones. He rushed to a nearby hospital emergency room in search of help. The pain was excruciating and he begged for relief. It was not forthcoming until after a series of events during which he signed a permission form for treatment, another for special X rays of his kidneys, and a third for an operation. Finally, he was given a strong pain medication and the pain began to ease. As he gradually fell under the influence of the drug, he was suddenly struck with panic. Though as an attorney he was trained to know better, he realized that in his desperate need for medical care he had signed three legal documents without even reading them.

Finally, you have completed your registration, and you can go to your room. Inside, you may sit on the bed wondering what to do next. Soon, an aide comes in and gives you a hospital gown. You ask what time your operation is going to be, but she says she doesn't know. After you change clothes, a nurse comes in and weighs you and checks your temperature, pulse, respirations, and blood pressure. You ask about your operation. She says that the doctor will be in later and to ask him. You begin to wonder about your right to be informed.

You sit down and wait. You begin to settle in, maybe read for a while. After a time, you step to the door and look down the long hall with its polished floors . . . be careful, they are the number one cause of accidents in hospitals. You wonder if you're allowed to venture out, but decide to wait. If you go down near the nursing station, you might get in the way of all those important medical activities. You wait some more, beginning to feel a little childish. You begin to wonder how to find always encourages his patients to choose the day they want to be discharged from the hospital. Invariably, he finds that patients show remarkable common sense about selecting a time to leave the hospital. Furthermore, patients go home much earlier than most doctors would have allowed. So, if you want to choose the time to go home and get away from the hospital, tell your doctor.

If your doctor insists you stay at the hospital, ask why. If the reasons seem to be logical medical contraindications, then you might decide to follow his advice. However, if they are just matters of convenience, or if the doctor is being overly protective, then insist upon going home. Most surgeons would be cooperative at that point and help you make the necessary arrangements. However, the question could develop into an issue. You might even be asked to sign a legal document releasing the doctors and the hospital from any liability in your case. Most patients are intimidated by such documents and either agree to stay in the hospital or sign the legal form.

But, remember, nurses are not policemen, doctors are not judges, and hospitals are not jails. You are entitled to walk out of the hospital and go home at any time you choose. The doctor may not like it, but after operating on you, he cannot abandon you until you are well. If you feel any problems or injustices about this, see your lawyer.

Once at home, you can take charge of your health again, eating those foods you know to be nutritious, maintaining a positive attitude, gradually increasing your exercise, and avoiding bad habits. You'll visit your doctor's office for suture removal and to be sure you are improving, but you should assume the responsibility for your own overall health. As you begin to feel well again and ready to resume where you left off, perhaps you'll realize that your life has been changed. It may seem as though your operation has had a far greater impact than just curing a disease that was amenable to surgery.

Many people have actually come through surgery with a new lease on life. Perhaps it's a rejuvenation of spirit, knowing they've survived a life-threatening experience, or maybe they've gained confidence from withstanding a serious stress. For whatever reason, many patients have discovered physical, mental, and spiritual vigor after undergoing surgery.

Perhaps you will see your surgery as a turning point. If your nutrition and exercise programs began with your preparation, you may also look upon surgery as a starting point for your continued health. Perhaps the programs of improved personal habits which helped you through surgery can also help you prevent disease in the future. If so, you may find that what you have learned as preoperative and postoperative care can enhance your whole life, helping you to be a happier, more productive person.

Imagine what a continued health program might do for you. After studying eleven thousand adults for five and a half years, the UCLA School of Public Health published their results. Seven criteria emerged as important simple health measures:

1)   Three nutritious meals a day
2)   Emphasis on breakfast
3)   Moderate exercise
4)   Seven or eight hours' sleep a night
5)   No smoking
6)   Moderate alcohol consumption
7)   Maintenance of moderate weight

The results showed that a thirty-five-year-old man who practiced three of these criteria had a life expectancy of sixty-seven years. One who practiced all seven, however, could expect to live to be seventy-eight. With just such a simple health plan, you could possibly add eleven years to your life.

Surgery can be a turning point for you. Certainly, it's good to know that your operation successfully cured your ailment. Furthermore, the health program you started in preparation and for postoperative care may actually prevent future disease so that you will never again find it necessary to go under the knife. More importantly, what you have learned from surgery may do more for your fulfillment of life than any operation could.

13

Surgery—Are You Ready for It?

. . . Chance favors only the mind that is prepared.

Louis Pasteur

Are you prepared now for the day you or your loved ones might need surgery? Certainly, you now know a lot more about surgery than ever before. You have looked at the historical development of surgery and how surgeons get to be the way they are. You have seen surgery both as a so-called science and as a business. You have a clear idea of the indications for surgery, and you know how to avoid unnecessary surgery. Furthermore, you have candidly thought about the risks, limitations, and complications—including death—and what you can do before and after an operation to help prevent those complications in your case.

You can plan step by step what to do if you are ever advised to have surgery, and you can come to a personal decision about your own operation and surgeon. You know about the benefits and risks of anesthesia, and with your understanding of pain and postoperative preventive techniques you can help yourself recuperate and return to good health.

On the other hand, when you face the prospect of surgery, you are subjected to a medical system which is far from perfect, one in which many doctors are judged to be incompetent, the number of malpractice suits is increasing dramatically, and the incidence of questionable practice is inestimable. To protect

133

your own interests and to exercise your right of free choice, you may have to become more involved in the decisions surrounding your own case. Attempts by the government and within the profession itself to improve the quality of medical care in the United States are not yet adequate to insure a level you might consider necessary for you and your family. Moreover, many people feel that the government cannot effectively regulate medical practice and that only a return to basic values within the profession itself can bring about a reversal of undesirable trends. Indeed, there are those who think that the need for so many controls simply indicates that the system itself should be fundamentally changed.

Agencies and organizations to protect you from incompetent and unscrupulous surgeons offer no guarantee. Medical and surgical societies are really educational guilds and political organizations and not even meant to protect you directly. The newer requirements set up by the Department of Health, Education and Welfare for peer review and second opinions may offer some help, but their total effect remains to be measured. Even the regulation of surgeons right in hospitals where the work is being done has not proved altogether effective; there is just too much cronyism, mutual protection of interests, and ineffeciency within regulatory committees. Of course, you can always resort to malpractice suits. But as a protective device for you or your family, even a successful malpractice lawsuit would give you only pyrrhic victory, because you can collect for damages only after the fact, after you or a loved one has suffered from negligence resulting in bodily injury or death. Collecting even millions of dollars to care for a paralyzed or crippled victim of malpractice is hardly what you hope to achieve from your medical care. How much better it would be if you took precautions and became informed beforehand.

Your knowledge about surgery can help you avoid those elements in the medical system that work against you. But aren't there also some ways you could actually help to change the system to make it work better for you, your family, and your community? Whatever your own interests or beliefs, you can have something to say about your health care through your elected representatives and by your own personal involvement.

In the United States Congress important health measure
being debated. Some politicians have been influenced by the
powerful lobbies of the American Medical Association, drug
companies, and health care industrialists. But the zeal of the
proponents of improved medical care has been dampened because of public apathy.

Although many people are aware of the injustices and dangers of the medical system, most just try to look out for themselves and their own families, protecting themselves by getting
health insurance, finding a doctor, and hoping for the best. But
the basic issues will not be solved until more people take an
active part in our American way of medicine.

What do you think about government programs for health
care? Would you like to continue present private insurance, institute a National Health Insurance, or adopt socialized medicine? Would you want to be assigned doctors or retain your
right of free choice? What can be done to improve medical practice? How can you stop unnecessary surgery and overutilization
of medical services? How can you help the medical profession
return to basic values? How can you ensure that that high-quali-
ty medical services are available to you?

When you stop to think about it, to be prepared for surgery
or any other medical services, you need to become more involved. Perhaps you should think more about the practice of
medicine and surgery in the United States and write to your
senator or congressperson. They can certainly use your opinions, and you might be surprised to see the effect you can have.

You can also influence your state government. Your property
and sales taxes support your medical schools. Your state representatives, governor, and other public officials have traditionally had a hands-off policy toward medical schools, leaving
the policies about admissions and curricula to the academic faculties.

Perhaps you would like your elected representatives to take a
more careful look at what's going on in your medical school.
Perhaps you would like to have something more to say about
who is admitted to your medical school, what the curriculum is,
and what kind of doctors will eventually be sent out into your
community. Perhaps you long for the days of the general practi-

tioner, when doctors seemed really to care about their patients.

Your state government also regulates the licensing of physicians. What is the quality of medical practice in your state? Are you protected by laws that require continuing education for doctor's and provide for stiff penalties when doctors behave unethically? Perhaps if you and your political organizations took these issues to your governor and state representatives, some changes might be instituted. You might be surprised to see how much you can influence medical education and practice in your state.

At the local level, you can be even more effective. If you ever need an operation, you can insist upon your rights. In one hospital, a woman patient was confronted with an operative permit for a breast biopsy. When she read the document, she discovered that she was also being asked to agree to a radical mastectomy if the biopsy turned out to be malignant. She refused, stating that she only wanted a biopsy and would think further about radical surgery after she knew the nature of the breast lump. The patient had read that such a procedure was acceptable medical treatment in most hospitals. However, the nurse became irritated, insisting that the patient sign the agreement. When the confrontation escalated, the nursing supervisor was called in, and she delivered an ultimatum that the patient either follow routine and sign the document or else they would cancel her operation and she could just go home. Facing this dilemma, the woman went to the phone and called her doctor at home, demanding her right to choose the method she preferred. Finally, the doctor agreed and came to the hospital to help make arrangements.

It might take a struggle, but if they know and insist upon their rights, patients can obtain the medical care they want. But it would be even better to prepare ahead of time. Perhaps you should find out about your hospital. What legal forms are patients required to sign? Who is the administrator? Who are the members of the board of trustees? Who sits on the executive committee? Who is the dietician? What is the hospital's accident rate? Is the hospital accredited? Through your civic service groups, volunteer organizations, and city or county government, you could probably help to improve your hospital. With enough enthusiasm, you might even find ways to install patient-consumer representatives on some of the committees. How about some new committees? A patient advocacy committee, or community advisory committee, or a human rights committee might do a lot to ensure that your hospital will be run with patients' interest paramount.

I hope that you are now prepared to face surgery. You know what you can do to protect yourself and to help yourself. Perhaps you even feel that your preparation and recuperation from surgery can help to enhance other aspects of your life. Moreover, maybe you are ready to exercise your right of representation in a democratic society to help bring surgery nearer its precious ideal of healing love.

14

Things You Should Know about Some Operations

No surgeon can discuss an operation to be performed upon you without first knowing every detail of your case and then getting to know you personally to learn about your beliefs, preferences, and fears. So, we will not try here to elucidate the details of anatomy, the vagaries of disease, or the many modifications of specific operations; there are just too many differences among individual patients and too many variations of particular surgical procedures to allow a general discussion that can be meaningful to every reader. If you are ever advised to have an operation, you should follow the steps outlined in Chapter Eight, asking your own doctors about every detail of your illness and the proposed therapy.

I would like to offer you some other important information about operations ... things you don't ordinarily hear from surgeons. I will emphasize some important and controversial aspects of indications, benefits, complications, alternatives, and your decision. After reading about these operations, you should be able to think about them critically, as surgeons do, and gain the insight to ask the most pertinent and incisive questions if surgery is ever recommended for you or your loved ones.

The following thirty-one general categories of operations comprise over 90 percent of major surgery performed in the United States:

Angiography (X Ray of Arteries and Veins)

Angiograms, X-ray pictures of arteries and veins, can be made by injecting contrast media into the bloodstream, then taking X rays of the circulation. Because these procedures are diagnostic they are often taken lightly by patients. But angiography is surgery.

Angiography involves inserting catheters into arteries and injecting foreign material into the bloodstream. It should be considered as carefully as any operation, judging the benefits and the potential risks. The operations are performed by cutting through the skin of the arm or groin and inserting long plastic catheters into the arteries. The tips of the catheters can then be positioned under a fluoroscope so that almost every artery of the body can be selectively studied by angiograms. Angiography is used most commonly to assess the circulation of the neck, the legs, and the heart itself, although selective studies of bowels, kidneys, liver, and other internal organs can be done.

You should keep in mind that angiograms are usually additional studies and ordinarily do not in themselves determine whether an operation should be performed. Terrible-looking angiograms can be obtained of organs that are functioning practically normally. However, after symptoms and examination indicate that an operation might be necessary, angiography can then be helpful to determine the feasibility and extent of surgery.

Less commonly, such as in crushing or penetrating trauma, angiograms may help to determine the necessity of an operation by demonstrating injuries of the blood vessels.

INDICATIONS:

The many various indications for arteriography or venography cannot be enumerated here. In general, these studies provide diagnostic information that cannot be obtained any other way.

1. Circulatory problems of the arms or legs manifested by pain, numbness, and loss of viability of the limb.

2. Circulatory problems of the arteries to the brain, manifested by mental confusion, dizziness, or intermittent "small strokes."

3. Circulatory problems of the coronary arteries, the vessels serving the heart itself.

4.   Crushing or penetrating injuries, which may have damaged arteries.

5.   Diagnostic problems such as tumors of the abdomen or chest when other less invasive methods fail to determine the nature of the lesions.

6.   Blood clots in veins can be diagnosed by angiography.

7.   Sites of hemorrhage within the abdomen or gastrointestinal tract can be located by angiography when other tests fail.

BENEFITS:

1.   Diagnosis of tumors of unknown origin.

2.   Diagnosis of injuries to blood vessels or other organs.

3.   Determination of feasibility or extent of operations on diseased arteries.

4.   Location of bleeding in the gastrointestinal tract.

COMPLICATIONS:

1.   Damage to arteries from the catheters resulting in loss of circulation and gangrene of the affected area.

2.   Local wound infection or hemorrhage.

3.   Sensitivity or allergic reactions to the contrast media, especially iodine, causing rashes, breathing difficulties, or circulatory collapse.

ALTERNATIVES:

1.   In some cases angiograms may offer so little additional diagnostic information, such as with swellings of arteries (aneurysms), that it may be better to proceed with operations without angiograms, especially in cases of emergency or possible sensitivity to iodine solutions.

2.   In other cases, angiogram may be unnecessary because an operation is inadvisable or patients refuse surgery beforehand.

3.   Newer noninvasive techniques, such as irradiation scanning, may supply the same or nearly the same information with less risk.

YOUR DECISION:

Be sure to ask questions about exactly what the tests involve and what it will mean for you. Obviously, if you don't want to have any further operations, then the angiograms aren't necessary. For instance, patients who prefer medical management instead of coronary bypass operations for heart disease do not need to have coronary angiograms of their hearts. Even if you are in favor of an operation, find out if other simpler tests can supply the same or nearly the same information. Incidentally, you might also want to ask what resuscitation equipment and competent doctors are available in the X-ray department in case you have a serious complication during your angiogram. You may even want to go to a different hospital if you find these safety features lacking.

Appendectomy

Even in some reputable hospitals, as many as 40 percent of appendectomies performed are done on normal appendixes. The symptoms and signs of disease that might have indicated possible appendicitis were instead proved to have been caused by some other illness, such as intestinal flu, lymph node inflammation inside the abdomen, or even pneumonia.

Undoubtedly, the number of appendectomies could be reduced. But the proponents for aggressive surgical approach say that not operating could be dangerous because then some real appendicitis could be missed, and ruptures might occur, causing a significant increase in the number of deaths. This philosophy is based on evidence reported in the 1930s, prior to antibiotics and some of the newer diagnostic techniques such as radiography scanning. Research to determine the usefulness of newer diagnostic and therapeutic techniques for appendicitis has not been done.

To date, only a careful approach to diagnosis and a scrupulous decision to operate can reduce the number of appendectomies. Sure, only one in a thousand or so patients die following appendectomy. If such deaths occur because of rupture of the appendix or spreading infection despite adequate surgical care, that is understandable. But if deaths occur in patients with normal appendixes for whom a more careful approach might have avoided the operation, that is tragic.

The diagnosis of appendicitis is very difficult. The utmost care and consideration must be given to patients with abdominal pain suggesting appendicitis.

INDICATIONS:

    1. A diagnosis of appendicitis.

    2. As a final diagnostic maneuver to determine whether a patient has acute appendicitis when the risk of spreading infection is especially dangerous or probable, such as in: infants; the elderly; pregnancy; underlying disease causing increased risk of infections, such as diabetes mellitus.

    3. Although controversial, appendectomy to prevent the possibility of appendicitis in the future is sometimes performed incidentally during other abdominal operations, such as gallbladder removal or hysterectomy.

BENEFITS:

    1. Appendectomy cures a source of infection inside the abdomen and prevents spread of the infection by rupture or by lymph channels or the bloodstream, problems which could lead to infection in other organs of the body, including the lungs, heart, liver, kidneys, brain, and bone.

    2. Removing the appendix incidentally during another operation can prevent an episode of appendicitis or any of its complications later in a patient's life.

    3. As a final diagnostic device, appendectomy provides the benefit of therapeutic appendectomy if the diagnosis is , indeed, appendicitis, and may also reveal other disease, such as abnormalities of the intestines, ovaries, or other abdominal or pelvic organs.

COMPLICATIONS:

    1. Unnecessary appendectomy because of eagerness to op-

erate rather than pursuing other means of diagnosis constitutes a major complication of the operation.

2. All the surgical and anesthetic complications described in Chapters Two and Six.

3. Complications such as adhesions or wound hernias can occur years after appendectomy.

ALTERNATIVES:

1. Watchful observation is usually advisable, especially if the diagnosis is not clear-cut. Sometimes, with a few hours' bed rest and repeat examinations and laboratory studies, operation becomes unnecessary. Only if the patient is "septic" with high fever and elevated white blood count or if rupture seems imminent is there need to rush into operation.

2. In doubtful cases, the diagnosis can sometimes be helped by special X Ray of the large intestine—barium enema.

3. Incidental appendectomy during another operation should not be taken lightly. It would be tragic if the primary operation went well and a complication was caused by removal of the normal appendix. Again, one must consider the risks versus possible benefits.

YOUR DECISION:

Considering the difficulty of diagnosis of appendicitis, your greatest concern before agreeing to appendectomy should be whether the diagnosis was made as carefully as possible. Obviously, the quality of your surgeon will be extremely important. Avoid another pitfall—sometimes when a family doctor, internist, or pediatrician decides upon a diagnosis of appendicitis, the surgeon is reluctant to disagree. In all cases, ascertain as best you can that the diagnosis was made with care. Is the history typical? Are the examination findings clear-cut? Have all the necessary laboratory tests been done? Is it advisable to have further tests, such as bowel X rays? Is it reasonable to wait for a few hours?

The mortality rate following appendectomy for unruptured appendixes is low, 0.1 percent. For ruptured appendicitis, the mortality is 3 percent, or 30 times as high. The statistics seem to weigh in favor of operating. However, some common sense is also in order and one must avoid making a decision out of fear. Although statistics aren't available, the risk of rupture in a patient without a clear-cut diagnosis is probably extremely small.

Whether to perform appendectomy routinely during other abdominal operations is controversial. Some surgeons prefer not to add unnecessary risks, however small. Others consider the risk so small as to warrant the prevention of appendicitis at a later date. Statistics aren't available. Fortunately, the risk of either option is small.

Arterial Surgery

Surgery to improve arterial circulation has been highly developed in the past twenty years. Arterial surgery can relieve pain, weakness, and subsequent gangrene resulting from blockage of arteries by arteriosclerosis. Although arterial surgery is performed mostly for disease of the legs, it can also improve blood flow in many arteries of the body, including those in the neck leading to the brain and those of the heart itself (see Coronary Bypass Operations). Sometimes the diseased arteries can be opened with careful dissection, but more often bypass procedures, using veins or artificial grafts made of woven dacron, are necessary to provide new condiuts through which blood can flow. Some surgeons now recommend more of these operations to improve circulation in elderly people suffering from arteriosclerosis.

INDICATIONS:

The indications for arterial surgery are based upon the patients' symptoms and the findings on physician examination. Pain in the calves or buttocks, for instance, can indicate blockage of the arteries to the legs. Mental confusion or dizziness can be caused by poor circulation through the arteries of the neck. Questioning about the exact nature of the symptoms and careful physical examination can determine if the circulation is impaired and whether operation upon the arteries is warranted. After an operation is deemed necessary, and the patient agrees, X rays (angiograms) are performed to see the exact architecture of the arteries and the extent of disease (see Angiography.)

BENEFITS:

1.   Relief of symptoms such as pain in the legs, angina pectoris, or mental signs of "small stroke."
2.   Improvement in circulation so that subsequent gangrene does not occur.
3.   The data supporting benefits from many arterial operations (especially those on neck arteries) are not statistically valid. Whether these operations are beneficial is open to question.

COMPLICATIONS:

1.   All the complications of major surgery and anesthesia discusses in Chapters Two and Six.
2.   Failure of the operations. Arterial surgery is fraught with a high incidence of failure, as high as 33 percent for some operations. Unfortunately, when these operations fail, circulation is worsened instead of improved, and gangrene or permanent paralysis usually results.
3.   System complications, such as heart attacks and strokes, occur with arterial surgery because arteriosclerosis is a generalized disease. During operations to fix one artery, blood loss or drug and anesthetic reactions can cause decreased circulation to other areas, such as the heart or brain. Careful evaluation is necessary to determine the overall health of patients who are to undergo arterial surgery.

ALTERNATIVES:

1.   Some patients get along without operations, reducing their activity to compensate for decreased blood flow.
2.   Some patients try medical treatments such as drugs to improve circulation.
3.   For patients who smoke, just stopping nicotine intake

and increasing exercise can greatly improve circulation, so that surgery is avoided.

YOUR DECISION:

Deciding about arterial surgery is difficult because once significant symptoms occur or impending gangrene becomes evident, some means to increase circulation must be instituted or the condition will certainly worsen. However, recognizing the high failure rates of arterial surgery and the questions regarding the efficacy of these operations, some patients may decide to wait, trying medical programs instead of running the risk of complications. All things considered, it is important to remember that arterial surgery is local treatment for a generalized, systemic disease.

Back Surgery

Back surgery performed to relieve curvature and injuries of the spine can be very useful. These special circumstances should be discussed thoroughly with the surgeons recommending the surgery.

Most back surgery is done for the relief of lower back pain and is controversial. Back pain can be caused by many different ailments, but most of it is due to strain, a condition that afflicts most people at some time during their lives. When pain becomes incapacitating, surgery is sometimes considered. Back surgery can be helpful for specific problems, such as ruptured intervetebral disc, but for ordinary back pain due to muscle strain, surgery rarely helps. Back operations are far from 100 percent effective, a fact to which many back pain sufferers will attest. At least some back operations are unnecessary and cannot hope for relief of pain.

INDICATIONS:

The indications for back operations vary widely from doctor to doctor. Some surgeons insist upon special X-ray studies of the spine (laminograms) to show without question that an oper-

able entity is present. Other surgeons operate without laminograms, and are satisfied when pain in the back seems typical.
These surgeons perform back operations more frequently. Their
rate of cure is less.

Sometimes, when sudden back pain strikes, the diagnosis of
ruptured disc can be made just with physical examination. In
these cases, most surgeons agree that an operation is urgent to
prevent damage to the nerve.

BENEFITS:

Relief of back pain so that people can perform their work and
enjoy recreation.

COMPLICATIONS:

1.   All the complications of surgery and anesthesia discussed
in Chapters Two and Six.
2.   Failure of the operation to relieve pain is the most frequent complication of back surgery.
3.   Damage to the nerve roots during operation can result in
permanent paralysis.
4.   Other complications resulting in nerve damage can result
from the special laminogram X rays of the back.

ALTERNATIVES:

1.   Continued medical management of pain using medication, heat, and whirlpool baths.
2.   Acupuncture, hypnosis, or meditation to relieve pain.
3.   Obtaining a referral to a pain clinic at a medical center or
VA hospital.
4.   Use of back exercises to strengthen the muscles of the
back, thereby relieving pain.

YOUR DECISION:

Lower back pain can be annoying, even exasperating. But
that in itself is not a good reason to have an operation. First,
patients should have some reasonable assurance that an opera-

tion will give relief. For some, the fact that their pain is the result of an industrial or military injury makes them feel they deserve relief and that an operation should be done. That is bad reasoning. Knowing about failures and the risks of surgery, patients might choose to continue medical management, adopting more aggressive attitudes toward relief of pain. Some could use back exercises more diligently. Others may try newer methods of pain control as discussed in Chapter Eleven.

Bone and Joint Operations

Many different bone and joint operations for the hips, knees, arms, legs, and ankles are available to relieve patients of debilitating pain, improve motion, and to enhance healing of fractures. For example, operations to place nails in hip fractures in elderly patients have increased life expectancy greatly by allowing early ambulation and exercise. Additionally, well-known football players and other athletes have had their careers improved greatly by knee and ankle operations.

Some operations on the joints can be overused, however, especially procedures designed to relieve symptoms. Removing cartilage from the knees of patients who have only minimal symptoms or are not particularly athletic, for instance, is unnecessary. The use of artificial elbows, hip, and knee joints is increasing rapidly. The indications for the placement of these artificial joints are not as yet well defined, and some of us wonder about the overuse of these expensive and risky operations, especially in elderly people, when lesser, more established procedures might give results nearly as good.

INDICATIONS:

1. When joint pain from severe arthritis or injuries is incapacitating.
2. In certain fractures when healing is unlikely or unreliable with casting or immobilization procedures.
3. When destruction of joints has occurred because of arthritis or injuries resulting in significant decrease in function.

BENEFITS:

1.   Improvement of healing of certain fractures.
2.   Improved comfort and function for individuals with incapacitating pain.
3.   Early ambulation instead of long-term traction, thereby preventing complications of prolonged bed rest, such as pneumonia or blood clots.

COMPLICATIONS:

1.   All the complications of surgery and anesthesia described in Chapters Two and Six.
2.   Failure to heal—sometimes the nails, clamps, and bone glues used for these operations actually interfere with healing.
3.   Infection of bone, osteomyelitis, is one of the most difficult diseases to cure. Usually, artificial joints, nails, or clamps must be removed for these infections to heal.

ALTERNATIVES:

For most surgery for bone and joints, nonoperative alternatives are available, and each particular case should be discussed thoroughly. For many bone and joint problems, some surgeons think surgery should not be undertaken until simpler, less risky methods have been tried. For example, some surgeons prefer casts or traction for fractures of the long bones of the arms or legs. For painful joints, many patients might get relief with medicine and physical therapy before hurrying into operations. Some patients might wish to try newer methods of pain control as discussed in Chapter Ten.

YOUR DECISION:

Knowing that not all of these operations are successful and recognizing the risk of surgery, you should consider all aspects of your particular case and all the alternatives before agreeing to operations on your bones or joints. Remember, surgery to relieve symptoms should be performed only if the patient feels the pain is incapacitating and cannot be relieved by simpler methods.

Bowel Surgery (Colon and Rectum)

Various operations are necessary for diseases of the colon and rectum. Frequently, these are performed to remove malignant tumors. Operations may also be required to remove certain benign tumors, polyps, depending upon their size and shape. When medical management fails, operations might also be required to treat inflammatory conditions of the large intestine, such as ulcerative colitis or diverticulitis.

When tumors or inflammation obstruct the colon, perforate through the wall of the bowel, or hemorrhage uncontrollably, emergency operations become necessary.

INDICATIONS:

1.   Cancer of the colon or rectum.
2.   Some benign polyps of the colon, which because they are large or irregularly shaped are suspicious of malignancy.
3.   Inflammation of the large intestine that does not respond to medical management.
4.   Obstruction, hemorrhage, or perforation of the colon for any reason.

BENEFITS:

1.   The possibility of cure of cancer. As high as 58 percent of colon cancers can be cured with surgery.
2.   Relief of symptoms due to inflammation, thereby improving digestion and nutrition.
3.   Repair of life-threatening conditions such as hemorrhage, obstruction, or perforation of the colon.

COMPLICATIONS:

1.   All the complications of surgery and anesthesia discussed in Chapters Two and Six.

2. Failure to heal can result in leaks from the intestine into the peritoneal cavity, resulting in spreading infection.

ALTERNATIVES:

1. In cases of cancer, there are few alternatives to colon and rectal surgery except to ascertain the full extensiveness of the disease and whether the operation offers a chance for cure.

2. The extensiveness of colon operations can vary, especially as to whether the rectum can be rejoined to provide normal bowel movements or if an artificial opening on the abdomen, a colostomy, is necessary.

3. Many polyps that once required major surgery can now be removed by an instrument used to look into the large bowel (colonoscope).

4. Even in cases of cancer of the rectum, some surgeons now advocate simple cauterization instead of extensive surgery.

YOUR DECISION:

Just knowing there might be alternatives to colon or rectal operations should encourage you to ask questions. In cases of benign polyps, you will certainly want to ask about colonoscopy before proceeding with major surgery. In cases of cancer, you will want to discuss the extensiveness of the procedure and especially to ask questions about colostomy. Additionally, before agreeing to an operation for inflammatory disease of the colon and rectum, you should carefully inquire as to the relative necessity of the operation and be sure that all measures for medical management have been tried before proceeding with major surgery.

Bowel Surgery (Small Intestine)

Various operations for inflammation or tumors of the small intestine are sometimes necessary. Most often, these operations are because of obstruction of the small intestine, which itself is usually caused by adhesions, scars in the peritoneal cavity that gradually constrict over the years until the small intestine is completely occluded and food can no longer pass. Hernias of the abdominal wall can entrap loops of small bowel causing obstruction (see Hernia Operations). Bowel obstructions can also be caused by clumps of food material that lodge in the intestine, occluding the passageway for food. This condition usually occurs in people who have had previous operations on their stomach and duodenum and who fail to chew their food thoroughly. In other cases, certain foods, such as persimmons, can actually harden inside the intestine producing small bowel obstruction. Certain inflammatory diseases of the bowel, such as Crohn's disease or tuberculosis, can also cause obstruction of the small intestine. Though rare, tumors of the small intestine can sometimes require operation.

INDICATIONS:

1.   Small bowel obstruction for any reason.
2.   Inflammatory disease of the small intestine that does not respond adequately to medical management.
3.   Tumors of the small intestine (rare).

BENEFITS:

Relief of small bowel obstruction allowing for return of normal digestion and nutrition. Repair of underlying disease such as hernia can also be accomplished.

COMPLICATIONS:

1.   All the complications of major surgery and anesthesia described in Chapters Two and Six.
2.   Recurrence—small bowel obstructions caused by adhesions frequently recur in months or years.

ALTERNATIVES:

Some small bowel obstructions secondary to adhesions will resolve with the use of long intestinal tubes, thereby avoiding major operations.

YOUR DECISION:

Operations on the small intestine are variable and each specific case should be discussed individually. However, just knowing that there might be alternatives should help you to ask more questions and to come to a personal decision before agreeing to an operation. For instance, you may want to ask about the use of long intestinal tubes rather than agreeing to an early operation for small bowel obstruction.

Breast Biopsy

Whether a lump in a woman's (or man's) breast should be removed for examination under the microscope can be a difficult decision. Most women have some benign cysts and nodules in their breast tissue. How does one decide which should be removed and examined for cancer? By physical examination alone, even experienced surgeons can tell in only about 70 percent of cases whether a breast lump is benign or malignant. Additional studies, such as X rays of the breast, mammograms and thermograms, can be helpful, but still, the only way to prove without question whether a breast lesion is benign or malignant is to examine the tissue under a microscope; and that means an operation—breast biopsy—to remove the lump. Rather than subjecting most of the female population to operations, however, it seems only logical to try to gather as much information as possible about each particular case, then proceed with surgery if it seems indicated.

Most breast biopsies are performed in operating rooms and the tissue is sent directly to pathology where it is quick-frozen so it can be sliced very thinly, then treated with special stains and examined under the microscope—a so-called frozen section. If a lump is proved by frozen section to be malignant, the surgeon will proceed with a cancer operation (see Breast Removal). Some studies have shown that removing breast lumps and waiting a day for the final diagnosis so that patients can decide carefully about further surgery gives cure rates as good as the frozen section technique.

INDICATIONS:

1. Breast lumps which by examination are hard, irregular in shape, or enlarging.
2. Breast lumps which on X ray or the thermogram studies show characteristics of malignancy.
3. Breast lumps in patients who worry, cannot sleep, and become emotionally distraught of the fear of cancer.

BENEFITS:

A definite diagnosis of questionable breast lesions and the effective treatment of cancer by early detection.

COMPLICATIONS:

1. All the complications of major surgery and anesthesia as discussed in Chapters Two and Six.
2. Misdiagnosis—rarely, false diagnoses of cancer have been made on frozen section and breasts have been removed unnecessarily.

ALTERNATIVES:

1. X-ray mammography or thermography are the primary alternatives prior to breast biopsy.
2. Watchful waiting with repeat examinations at intervals can sometimes help determine that a lump is benign.
3. Self-examination may be the best way to determine the nature of breast lumps. By getting to know the "map" of their own breasts, women can recognize the lumps and cysts. A lump that has been present for years, even if discovered by a doctor on examination, is probably not malignant. On the other hand, a lump that has been present for years but is starting to enlarge is highly significant.
4. Some cysts of the breast can be "aspirated," the fluid inside removed by needle and syringe. If the cyst doesn't recur, there is no need for biopsy.

YOUR DECISION:

Careful judgment is required to determine if breast biopsy is necessary. Your self-examination can be a very helpful part of the evaluation. If you see a surgeon and he readily recommends biopsy, ask what the criteria are which make immediate operation necessary, then obtain a second opinion.

Remember, if you choose frozen section technique, you should know all about the operation that might be performed if the lump turns out to be malignant. That means a careful evaluation of all the statistics and choices about each of the operations for breast cancer.

Careful evaluation and judgment are required for women with lumps in their breasts. All women should obtain information from the American Cancer Society and their doctors and think about the possibility of breast biopsy and malignancy.

Breast Removal (Mastectomy)

Surgery of the breast is controversial and deserves the careful consideration of all women. The traditional operation for cancer of the breast, radical mastectomy, includes removing the entire breast, the contents of the armpit and the underlying pectoral muscles. More recently, some specialists have pointed out that cancer of the breast never spreads to the pectoral muscles. They have developed a modified operation in which the pectoral muscles are spared. Other surgeons reasoned that X-ray treatments could greatly improve some cancer of the breast, and they advocated only simple removal of the breast tissue without removing either the underlying muscles or doing a meticulous dissection of the armpit. They have reported results with simple mastectomy and irradiation as good as with radical surgery. Still other surgeons advocate not removing the breast at all, but instead taking out the malignant tissue with a surrounding normal border and following up with X-ray treatments. They also can show results as good as with radical surgery. Many combinations of these procedures for various types and extensiveness of breast cancer have also been tested.

Surgeons argue vehemently about these various modes of therapy, and advocates of the various procedures can all quote masses of scientific data to support their own points of view. Obviously, you cannot hope to study all the conflicting analyses. However, you should know that these choices are available and learn all about your own case in terms of which treatment you might prefer. Thorough consultation with your doctors about these choices is exceedingly important before you agree to any operation for cancer of the breast.

Some surgeons have even recommended removal of the breasts to prevent cancer in those women who might be prone to malignancy, such as women in families with high cancer rates or for precancerous inflammatory conditions of the breast, mastitis. These operations involve removal of the breast tissue, leaving the skin intact, and then placing artificial implants to retain the normal contour and texture of the breasts. These operations are controversial.

INDICATIONS:

1. Malignant lesions of the breast proven by biopsy (see Breast Biopsy).
2. "Precancerous" mastitis (controversial).

BENEFITS:

Overall cure of 55 percent and up to 80 percent cure for certain cancers of the breast. Whether one operative technique is better than others is still unknown.

COMPLICATIONS:

1. All of the complications of surgery and anesthesia discussed in Chapters Two and Six.
2. Occasional uncontrollable swelling of the arm occurs when dissection of the armpit has been performed.
3. Psychological disturbances often follow amputation of any part of the body. These emotional disturbances can be especially severe following breast removal.

4. Many complications of X-ray therapy occur following treatment for breast cancer, including pneumonia, bone marrow damage, injury to adjacent tissues, and varying degrees of general malaise associated with radiation.

5. Recurrence of cancer, either in the area of operation or by spreading to other parts of the body.

ALTERNATIVES:

Once cancer of the breast has been diagnosed, surgery to one degree or another together with X-ray treatments and possibly hormone therapy is usually advisable. However, the extensiveness of surgery varies widely.

YOUR DECISION:

The decision as to which operation to have for cancer of the breast is difficult. Just knowing about the choices, however, should help you to ask questions about your own case. You might prefer the simpler procedures, reasoning that the results are as good as more radical operations and you can keep your breasts intact. On the other hand, you might decide on a more radical approach, preferring extensive resection of cancer from your body. The important thing is to know the alternatives and come to a personal decision after careful consideration of all possibilities.

Cancer Operations

Cancer should be thought of not as one disease but as a general category of many different diseases. Consequently, patients must discuss their own particular case with their own doctors. However, surgery offers primary and adjunct treatment of most cancer. Removal of cancerous lesions of the lungs, stomach, intestinal tract, kidneys, and other organs constitutes definitive treatment for most lesions. Even for cancers in which the primary treatment is with irradiation or medicines, surgery offers additional treatment, such as bone-marrow transplants as adjunctive therapy for leukemia. Because of surgery, cure rates of over 90 percent can be achieved for many patients with cancer, and even when there isn't a chance for cure surgery can prolong life and improve the quality of life for some.

However, the surgical treatment of cancer is not altogether clear-cut. Doctors disagree sharply about many questions. For instance, some surgeons do not recommend operations for thyroid cancer anymore, pointing out that medical management gives results as good as surgery (see Thyroid Surgery). For other cancer, such as breast and stomach, doctors disagree about how extensive surgery should be (see Breast Removal and Ulcer Operations, Stomach). Furthermore, X-ray therapy for some cancer, such as certain tumors of the cervix and some skin and lip lesions, gives results as good as does surgery.

INDICATIONS:

1. Cancer in which there is a chance of cure.
2. Cancer that cannot be satisfactorily treated by other means.
3. As palliation, to improve the patient's condition even if the cancer itself is incurable.
4. As an adjunct to medical treatment of cancer.

BENEFITS:

1. Cure of cancer.
2. Improvement in life span and quality of life.

COMPLICATIONS:

1. All the complications of surgery and anesthesia discussed in Chapters Two and Six.
2. Many other complications specific to particular operations.

ALTERNATIVES:

Patients should discuss alternatives to their own specific condition before accepting surgery, inquiring about possible medical management and the extensiveness of proposed operations.

YOUR DECISION:

Just knowing about alternatives should encourage you to ask questions about your own specific problem if you are ever advised to have an operation for cancer. Unfortunately, the word *cancer* evokes feelings of fear and despair in many people. However, recognizing the possible benefits and complications of surgery, you should investigate and carefully decide about what treatment you might want for cancer.

Cataract Removal

Cataracts, opacities in the lenses of the eyes, can obstruct vision to varying degrees. Rarely, cataracts occur congenitally in young people, but the great majority are an affliction of age. When the opacities decrease vision, interfering with work or recreation, the lenses can be removed surgically, thereby allowing light into the eyes again. Thus, with the aid of special glasses or artificial lenses inserted into the eyes, vision is improved.

Though improved, vision after cataract removal is not the same as it was before the disease occurred. Images seem larger, and although central vision is better, peripheral vision is not good.

INDICATIONS:

1. Some eye doctors believe that a definite improvement in the quality of life or ability to earn a living should be reasonably obtainable if cataract surgery is to be done. Other doctors think that all cataracts should be removed when discovered.

2. Obviously, if systemic illness, nerve impairment, or retinal disease is the cause of visual difficulties, cataract removal will not help.

3. Most eye doctors recommend a personalized approach, carefully evaluating each individual patient before deciding about cataract removal.

BENEFITS:

Improved vision. Some patients can increase their ability to earn a living because of improved vision. Retired people can participate in recreation and travel. Even sedentary individuals can enjoy reading and watching television and movies.

COMPLICATIONS:

    1.   Hemorrhage is rare, but can result in blindness.
    2.   Infection is also rare, but can also cause blindness.
    3.   Glaucoma—1 or 2 percent of patients will develop glaucoma later.
    4.   Retinal detachment—1 or 2 percent of patients will develop a later retinal detachment.
    5.   Failure to achieve the desired results. Patients should be carefully advised beforehand as to what to expect in the way of visual improvement so they do not have unrealistic expectations.

ALTERNATIVES:

The alternative is to wait, and to learn to live with impaired vision. On the other hand, cataract surgery is making great advances, and you may wish to investigate the techniques, such as artificial lens implants.

YOUR DECISION:

Be sure to learn all about your cataracts and what the operation might have to offer you. If your vision is pretty good, you may want to avoid the risks and live with what you have. You will need all the facts about your own case before you can decide.

Coronary Bypass Surgery

Coronary bypass operations are designed to provide blood flow around arteriosclerotic occlusions of the coronary arteries, the vessels that serve the heart muscle itself. Veins are transplanted from the leg, one end sewn into the aorta, the main artery of the chest, and the other end into the coronary arteries themselves. The procedure involves open-heart surgery during which the patient's heart and lung functions are performed by a machine. The operations are a technical triumph and are coming into widespread use.

The research supporting the efficacy of these operations is still incomplete. Some doctors feel that coronary bypass operations should remain experimental until the procedures have been proved beyond any doubt to be effective. Thus far, the data are incomplete. Certainly, some patients have benefited dramatically, obtaining relief of chest pain, decreasing potent heart medications, and reducing the necessity of frequent hospitalizations. Other patients, however, have died on the operating table, never awakening from the anesthetic. Still others have been disappointed when their operations have failed to achieve relief of heart symptoms. Furthermore, not only are these operations sometimes ineffective, data are just beginning to be reported about the recurrence of symptoms for those patients who initially had good results from surgery. The recurrence rate has been termed "alarming" by reputable doctors. Even for those patients who do not suffer repeat heart attacks, the recurrence of severe chest pain and return to heart medications has been reported at an annual rate of 7 percent. This latest figure adds to the quandary of whether for all patients and for long-term results coronary bypass operations are actually beneficial.

INDICATIONS:

1. Heart attacks, myocardial infarctions, after which angiograms demonstrate localized lesions of one or more coronary arteries.

2. Incapacitating chest pain of heart origin, angina pectoris.

3. Some investigators are beginning to advocate coronary bypass operations for patients with even mild symptoms of heart disease.

BENEFITS:

The benefits are questionable. Thus far, coronary bypass operations have not been proved either to prevent recurrent heart attacks or to prolong life. They decrease the frequency and severity of chest pain in a certain percentage of patients. However, a careful report by a renowned cardiologist shows that good modern medical management of heart disease gives results as good as surgery for most types of coronary artery disease.

COMPLICATIONS:

1.   Death on the operating table or shortly thereafter. This has been reported as high as 5.6 percent in some reputable studies, although other surgeons claim percentages nearer 2 or 3 percent.
2.   All the complications of major surgery and anesthesia described in Chapters Two and Six.
3.   Unusual cases of mental confusion and intermittent psychosis following open-heart surgery.
4.   Failure of the operation to relieve symptoms.
5.   Recurrence of heart disease symptoms at a later date.

ALTERNATIVES:

Careful, thorough, and up-to-date management of heart disease.

YOUR DECISION:

Knowing that medical management has shown promising results, you should carefully consider the risks of undergoing an operation that has not been proved beyond a doubt to be more effective than more conservative methods of treating heart disease. Since at least some reports show medical management to be as good as surgery you may decide to continue care under an internist or cardiologist. Remember, if you don't want heart surgery, then you also don't need coronary angiograms (see

Angiography). It may be difficult to refuse an operation that is becoming more or less the standard mode of therapy, but remember that other once-popular heart operations have been discontinued after more careful evaluation.

On the other hand, you may welcome the chance to undergo an operation that might improve your heart condition. After all, some surgeons have undergone the operation themselves, and everyone must decide for themselves after learning all the facts.

Cosmetic Surgery

Augmenting small breasts, reducing large breasts, stretching out wrinkles, enlarging buttocks, removing fat, changing noses and chins . . . these are all the province of cosmetic surgery. More serious "reconstructive" surgery is called for to repair the ravages of war, fire, accidents, etc. The services can be obtained in most cities and towns, sometimes performed by certified plastic surgeons and other times by doctors without the sanction of the plastic surgical societies. All of these doctors offer techniques at various prices for those who wish or need to enhance their personal appearance.

INDICATIONS:

Purely the choice of individuals.

BENEFITS:

Individual benefits ranging from improved personal feeling of desirability and confidence to increased ability to earn a living.

One man was able to get a job in the youth-oriented advertising field once he'd had his face lifted. A woman had burn scars on her hands removed so she could go into company without embarrassment. People undergo cosmetic transformations for many reasons, often to overcome a deep sense of inferiority. The change in appearance enhances their sense of well-being and often leads to a more contented life.

COMPLICATIONS:

1.   All the complications of surgery and anesthesia discussed in Chapters Two and Six.

2.   Failure to achieve the anticipated results can be because of complications, but it can occur also because of unrealistic expectations.

3.   Sometimes cosmetic surgery results in serious disappointment leading to physical and emotional consequences of far-reaching importance.

ALTERNATIVES:

Unless cosmetic surgery is needed to overcome serious scarring, disfiguration, and/or emotional problems, individuals might also seek out beauticians and make-up artists to achieve new effects. There are also minor surgical procedures such as dermabrasion of the skin.

YOUR DECISION:

Recognizing that there is no guarantee of good cosmetic results and that there is some chance of untoward consequences or other complications, you would be wise to consider all aspects of cosmetic surgery before seeking it.

D & C (Diagnostic, Therapeutic, and for Abortion)

D & C stands for *dilatation and curretage,* a gynecological operation to dilate the opening (cervix) of the womb (uterus), and to suction or scrape out the contents. The procedure can be diagnostic, to remove and examine under the microscope the lining of the uterus. It can also be therapeutic, to help regulate the menstrual cycle, to resolve fertility problems, and to perform an abortion.

INDICATIONS:

1.   Suspicion of cancer of the lining of the uterus.

2.   To regulate menstrual cycles.

3.   To increase fertility for patients who have difficulty getting pregnant.

4.   To perform abortions.

5.   To control hemorrhage from any cause, such as retained tissue following childbirth, partial miscarriages, or incomplete surgical abortions.

BENEFITS:

1.   Early diagnosis and possible cure for uterine cancer.

2.   Regulation of menstrual cycles.

3.   Control of bleeding from the uterus.

4.   Lifesaving abortions for patients who cannot tolerate the stress of pregnancy because of serious illness.

5.   Birth control and family planning (depending upon individual beliefs and preferences).

COMPLICATIONS:

1.   Perforation of the uterus.

2.   Severe hemorrhage.

3.   All the complications of surgery and anesthesia discussed in Chapters Two and Six.

4.   Emotional reactions following gynecological operations. Patients who suffer guilt about abortion are especially prone to depression following D & C.

ALTERNATIVES:

1.   Hormonal control of some menstrual irregularities and fertility problems.

2.   Other methods of birth control or family planning.

3.   Other ways to deal with unwanted pregnancy such as having the baby and offering it for adoption.

YOUR DECISION:

The use of D & C for gynecological disease can be very helpful. You should ask about the necessity of D & C in your own particular case and whether less invasive methods might accomplish the same goals.

Abortions are controversial, involving philosophical and religious beliefs. Recognizing possible complications, especially emotional problems, patients should think carefully before submitting to abortion, seeking advice from their loved ones, women's organizations, Planned Parenthood or religious counselors.

Endoscopy (Special Internal Examinations)

Various "scopes" have been used for years to look into the bronchial tubes, the urinary bladder, and the lower colon and rectum. Doctors have even developed a peritoneoscope, an instrument that can be inserted through a small incision on the abdomen to inspect the internal organs. Not only can doctors see inside patients with these instruments, but operations can be performed through them, such as biopsy of the lung, removal of prostate gland, removal of colon polyps, biopsy of cancers of the lower colon and rectum, and tubal ligation for female sterilization (see Tubal Ligation). Since the development of fiberoptics, images can be transmitted along flexible plastic tubes, and even more useful scopes have been invented to diagnose and treat lesions of the esophagus and stomach (gastroscope), the entire length of the colon (colonoscope), the inside of joints (arthroscope). With special equipment some investigators are even looking inside arteries, the bile ducts, and the ventricles of the brain.

Endoscopy can be very useful, providing diagnostic information and therapeutic manipulations that would otherwise require major surgery. By helping to identify the nature of tumors, for instance, they can prevent major operations of the colon and urinary bladder. Furthermore, by helping to locate sites of bleeding and to identify other lesions, endoscopy can greatly improve the possibility of success of later surgery.

But the indications for the use of these instruments are not yet clearly defined, and undoubtedly some endoscopy now performed is unnecessary. Obviously, most patients with simple constipation or indigestion do not need endoscopy. Furthermore, some lesions such as duodenal ulcers can be identified by X ray and do not require further examination by endoscopy.

INDICATIONS:

1.   Locating sources of disease within the body that cannot be identified with less invasive methods, such as direct examination, X ray, or radioactive scanning.
2.   Relief of certain large bowel obstructions.
3.   Identification and control of internal bleeding.
4.   Differentiation between malignant and benign tumors.
5.   Definitive operations such as colon polyp removal, prostate operations, and tubal ligations.

COMPLICATIONS:

1.   All the complications of surgery and anesthesia discussed in Chapters Two and Six.
2.   Perforations of internal organs. Usually major surgery is necessary to repair the damage.
3.   Drug reactions—endoscopy is often performed on patients given high doses of strong medications. Serious reactions can occur.

ALTERNATIVES:

Other noninvasive and less dangerous methods can sometimes provide the same information.

YOUR DECISION:

You should ask questions if endoscopy is ever advised for you. Remember, these diagnostic tests are in themselves major operations and fraught with complications. Can the same information be obtained in a less dangerous, noninvasive method? Is the information sought after really necessary? Is there a more commonsense approach to minor symptoms such as constipation or indigestion? Recognizing that there are distinct risks, you should ascertain the necessity of endoscopy for you.

Gallbladder Operations (Cholecystectomy)

Most surgeons agree that all diseased gallbladders should be removed, even if the symptoms they produce are minimal, unless the patient's health is so poor that an operation would be life-threatening. Their reasoning is based upon autopsy studies that show that a certain number of people die every year as a result of complications of gallbladder disease who might have been spared if they had been operated upon at an earlier date.

No statistically valid research has been done, however, to demonstrate clearly in which patients the risk of operation might be greater than the risk of the disease. If a patient is overwhelmed with infection, if a gallbladder is about to rupture, if gallstones are blocking the flow of bile and causing jaundice, or if indigestion from gallbladder attacks is incapacitating, the necessity to operate seems rather obvious. On the other hand, a ninety-five year-old patient with severe heart disease and only mild indigestion secondary to gallstones probably wouldn't benefit from an operation.

Between those extremes, different patients suffer varying severity of gallbladder symptoms and are in different states of general health. Consequently, some doctors prefer to individualize treatment, first trying to determine if the severity of gallbladder symptoms is worth the risk of possible complications of an operation. For instance, some gastroenterologists think that patients past the age of fifty-five should not have gallbladder removal if their symptoms are minimal. This advice is given much to the chagrin of most surgeons, who say that waiting for gallbladder removal can only lead to more serious trouble later. The controversy goes on, and you will have to decide for yourself after asking lots of questions, if you are ever advised to have your gallbladder removed.

During gallbladder operations, nearby organs, especially the main bile ducts from the liver, are examined to determine the extent of disease and to make corrections when necessary. Some surgeons also perform special X-ray studies, injecting radiographic contrast media into the bile ducts to obtain pictures of the channels. Under certain circumstances, the bile ducts might actually be opened and inspected carefully within to insure that disease is not present or to correct any abnormalities found. These practices are fairly standard, but some variations from surgeon to surgeon do exist.

Diagnosis of gallbladder disease prior to surgery can sometimes be difficult. Sometimes a diseased gallbladder is easily identifiable on X-ray studies, stones or other abnormalities clearly visible. Other times, however, the evidence for gallbladder disease is presumptive, based upon the evidence that the gallbladder fails to visualize on X ray after the appropriate pills and preparation are given. However, care must be taken to insure that the gallbladder test X ray is done properly. If patients vomit or have diarrhea after taking the pills, or if there is liver or other disease present, then the gallbladder might not visualize even though it is normal. The diagnostic tests must be performed carefully to be a reliable index of gallbladder disease.

INDICATIONS:

1. Acute inflammation manifested by fever and pain in the right upper abdomen under the rib cage.
2. Chronic inflammation resulting in varying degrees of indigestion.
3. Stones in the gallbladder causing symptoms.
4. Doctors do not agree about stones that do not cause symptoms.
5. Various benign or malignant tumors (rare).

BENEFITS:

1. Prevention of progression of disease or complications caused by gallstones entering the main bile ducts or eroding through the gallbladder wall into other organs.
2. Relief or prevention of recurrence of inflammation and infection within the body.

3.   Relief of indigestion.

COMPLICATIONS:

1.   All the complications of surgery discussed in Chapters Two and Six.
2.   Unnecessary operations for normal gallbladders because of inadequate X-ray studies.
3.   Leakage of bile in the operative area, producing an abscess under the liver.
4.   Hemorrhage in the operative area.
5.   Injury to the bile ducts during operation. This complication is not uncommon, and is caused by less than optimal technique during surgery. Complicated operations are necessary to relieve the resultant bile leaks or later obstruction of the bile ducts.

ALTERNATIVES:

1.   Many surgeons recommend immediate operation when suddenly acute inflammation of the gallbladder occurs. Other surgeons prefer a less dramatic approach since most acute inflammation of the gallbladder can be relieved in a few days using stomach tube drainage, antibiotics, antispasmodics, and fluid replacement. Surgeons tend to recommend their own choices as to early or later operations. But only if the gallbladder is markedly enlarged and seems likely to rupture, or if there is spreading infection, is there need to operate immediately.
2.   Patients with only mild symptoms may prefer not to have a gallbladder operation unless the disease worsens. These patients may find relief simply by following a prescribed low-fat diet.
3.   Repeating gallbladder X rays if the diagnosis is based upon presumptive evidence of nonvisualization may be advisable, especially if any other cause for nonvisualization is suspected.

YOUR DECISION:

1.   Be sure the diagnosis has been made correctly before you decide.

2. Remember, in cases of acute attacks, you have a choice about whether to have an urgent operation or to wait for the inflammation to subside and decide later about surgery, after you have learned more about your illness, the proposed operation, and, of course, your choice of surgeons.

3. Think carefully about whether to have your gallbladder removed if you do not have severe symptoms. Remember, doctors disagree about this and you may want to make up your own mind after becoming thoroughly informed about your own case.

4. Ask whether your symptoms might be caused by some problem other than gallbladder disease.

5. Weigh the benefits versus the risks and then decide.

Hemorrhoidectomy

Almost all hemorrhoidectomies would be unnecessary if patients knew how to take proper care of their hemorrhoids to prevent symptoms (see Chapter Five).

1. Retrain your bowel habits, never straining at stool, but instead allow normal natural reflexes to take over the function of defecation.

2. Learn to respond to natural urges to have bowel movements rather than letting work or social distractions delay normal defecations.

3. Keep stools at a normal consistency, not too soft and not too hard, by proper fiber diet and occasional use of gentle laxatives.

4. Use a hot cloth instead of paper to clean the anus after bowel movement.

5. Use hot baths to cleanse and soothe the anus at the first signs of itching or burning of hemorrhoids.

6. Use some of the commercially available hemorrhoid preparations when itching or burning flares.

INDICATIONS:

1. Rarely, gangrene, infection, or severe bleeding may necessitate hemorrhoid operations.

2. Patients should decide for themselves about hemorrhoidectomy after carefully trying simpler methods.

BENEFITS:

Relief of symptoms of hemorrhoids.

COMPLICATIONS:

1. All the complications of surgery and anesthesia described in Chapters Two and Six.
2. Strictures of the anus because of scarring, requiring dilatations or corrective surgery.

ALTERNATIVES:

1. Grin and bear it.
2. Resolve to take better care of your hemorrhoids.
3. Exercise, such as jogging, is good for hemorrhoids. Some runners have found marked improvement in their hemorrhoids after beginning exercise programs.

YOUR DECISION:

Just knowing that hemorrhoidectomy can be unnecessary should give you a completely free choice about the operation. Remember, you should weigh the possible benefits versus the alternatives and risks before deciding to undergo this elective surgery.

Hernia Operations (Abdominal Wall Hernias)

Hernias, sometimes called ruptures, occur at areas of weakness of the abdominal wall, such as the groin, the umbilicus, or in scars of previous operations. In some patients, the muscles and fibrous tissue in these weak areas actually separate and allow internal organs such as the intestine to protrude under the skin enclosed in a sac composed of the inner lining of the abdominal cavity. The swelling of hernias can produce pain and discomfort. Sometimes, internal organs can get stuck outside the abdomen, incarcerated in the hernia sac. If untreated, incarceration can produce pressure on the enclosed organs, resulting in gangrene.

Beltlike devices, trusses, have been developed to reduce the bulging of hernias and to hold the internal organs inside the abodmen where they belong. More frequently, though, hernias are treated by surgical repair.

INDICATIONS:

Most surgeons recommend that any hernia of the groin should be repaired when discovered or soon thereafter. They point out that approximately four thousand deaths occur annually because of strangulated hernias. However, most of those deaths are of individuals who do not take care of themselves, and no one knows what the risk is to those who choose not to have hernia operations but instead wear fitted trusses and carefully watch for any signs of incarceration.

Umbilical hernias occurring in newborns should not be operated upon immediately; most of them heal themselves by the age of two years. In adults, however, elective repair of umbilical hernia is usually recommended.

When hernias become incarcerated and despite all maneuvers cannot be reduced back into the abdomen, urgent operation becomes necessary because of the obstruction of bowel and the possibility of gangrene. Certain hernias in females, near the major arteries and nerves to the legs (femoral hernias), should be repaired without undue delay because of the high incidence of incarceration.

BENEFITS:

Hernia operations relieve swelling and pain, thereby providing increased comfort and freedom of movement, especially for those people who perform heavy work or participate in athletics. Furthermore, these operations prevent hernias from becoming worse or developing incarceration or other problems later.

COMPLICATIONS:

1.   All the complications of surgery and anesthesia discussed in Chapters Two and Six.

2.   Recurrence of hernias months or years following surgery requires even more extensive operations.

ALTERNATIVES:

Wearing trusses can be satisfactory for some patients, especially those who do not do heavy work or participate in vigorous exercise. Care must be taken, however, to observe for pain or inflammation signaling incarceration.

After deciding about surgery for hernias, patients should next consider how the operation will be done. Most often, hernias are repaired under general or spinal anesthesia and patients are kept in the hospital for a few days. However, if you wish, you can probably find a surgeon who can repair your hernia under local anesthesia, and you can go home a few hours after the operation, thus avoiding the risks of anesthesia and prolonged hospitalization.

YOUR DECISION:

Knowing about the benefits, risks, and alternatives, you can decide if, when, and how you prefer to have an operation for your hernia.

Hiatus Hernia Operations

Hiatus hernias are protrusions of portions of the stomach up into the chest through a weak area on the diaphragm where the foodpipe (esophagus) passes though. More than 30 percent of people have small hiatus hernias. Almost all of them experience no symptoms or only occasional mild discomfort and do not need any treatment. For those few people who develop more bothersome symptoms, such as heartburn or difficulty swallowing, medical programs similar to ulcer treatment to reduce the acid in the stomach are satisfactory. For others, more vigorous programs, elevating the heads of their beds to prevent regurgitation of stomach acid up into the esophagus and following strict, bland diets, might be necessary. For those few patients with severe symptoms whom careful medical management fails to give relief, operations are sometimes recommended.

For years, internists have argued with surgeons about how severe symptoms should be before performing hiatus hernia operations. Surgeons argue with one another about which particular operations should be used. Some surgeons advocate repair through the chest; others, the abdomen. Many different operations have been developed for hiatus hernia repair, all with varying degrees of success and complication rates.

INDICATIONS:

1. Incapacitating symptoms of hiatus hernia.
2. Severe ulcerations or strictures of the lower esophagus.
3. Rarely, hemorrhage, perforation, or even gangrene in hiatus hernias can require emergency operations.

BENEFITS:

1. Relief of indigestion.
2. Cure of lesions of the lower esophagus.
3. Lifesaving cure for hemorrhage or perforations.

COMPLICATIONS:

1. All the complications of surgery and anesthesia discussed in Chapters Two and Six.
2. Failure to achieve results—sometimes symptoms persist despite hiatus hernia repair.
3. Recurrence of hernias at a later date.
4. Misdiagnosis—sometimes symptoms attributed to hiatus hernia are really caused by other problems, such as heart disease. In such cases, hiatus hernia operations are obviously ineffective.

ALTERNATIVES:

1.   More vigorous medical management of symptoms of hiatus hernia.

2.   More careful diagnostic evaluation to determine the exact cause of symptoms.

YOUR DECISION:

If a hiatus hernia operation is ever recommended for you, be sure to assess for yourself the severity of your symptoms and whether possible benefits are worth the risks. Also, ask if your symptoms might be caused by some other ailment. Then learn about the operation, its rates of cure, recurrence, and complications.

Hysterectomy

Hysterectomy is an operation to remove the uterus with or without the attached Fallopian tubes and ovaries. The operation can be performed through the abdomen or through the vagina. Nearly a million hysterectomies are performed annually in the United States. Many of them are unnecessary (see Chapter Five).

INDICATIONS:

The indications for hysterectomy vary from doctor to doctor depending upon various philosophies. Some surgeons believe that the uterus should be removed after childbearing years as a measure to prevent cancer from occurring at a later date. Others feel that hysterectomy should be performed only for definite indications such as cancer.

DEFINITE INDICATIONS:

1.   Most cancer of the cervix or uterus.
2.   Large benign tumors, such as fibroids, which produce

symptoms of pressure and pain in the pelvis.
    3. Chronic, uncontrollable infections of the uterus.
    4. Uncontrollable hemorrhage.

CONTROVERSIAL INDICATIONS:

    1. Sterilization.
    2. Prevention of later disease.
    3. Small, benign tumors or cysts.
    4. Ovarian cysts.
    5. Enlarged uterus.
    6. Tipped uterus.
    7. Vague pelvic pain or discomfort.
    8. Irregular menstrual periods.

BENEFITS:

Relief of symptoms, cure of cancer, prevention of cancer, and sterilization.

COMPLICATIONS:

    1. All the complications of surgery and anesthesia discussed in Chapters Two and Six.
    2. Technical errors—especially inadvertent cutting of the ureter, the tube from the kidney to the bladder.
    3. Psychological depression.
    4. Uncontrollable symptoms of surgical menopause if ovaries are removed.

ALTERNATIVES:

    1. Some cancer of the cervix can be treated with X ray (see Cancer Operations).
    2. Periodic Pap smear and pelvic examination for cancer.
    3. Less drastic methods of birth control.
    4. Hormone therapy for menstrual disorders.

YOUR DECISION:

Recognizing the wide disagreements among gynecologists

themselves over the indications for hysterectomy, you should ask lots of questions about your own particular case and find out what the doctors are arguing about so that you can make up your own mind. Bearing in mind that some women have died from the complications of hysterectomy, you might want to try other methods of achieving your goals, whether they are to prevent cancer or to provide birth control.

In cases of cancer, you should discuss carefully all the aspects of your particular case and find out about the feasibility of other treatments.

If you are going to have a hysterectomy, be sure to discuss all the aspects of the operation with your surgeon. Ask about the problems of surgical menopause symptoms, and decide how extensive you want your operation to be.

Kidney Stone Operations

Some kidney stones are practically harmless and hardly interfere with normal function. But when stones try to exit from the kidney down the long thin tubes (ureters) that lead to the bladder, trouble begins. The stones are just a little too large for the ureters, and excruciating pain results. Even so, most stones will successfully travel down the ureters into the bladder, then pass with urination outside the body. Occasionally, stones become lodged in the ureters, unable to pass into the bladder. That is when surgery to remove them becomes necessary.

INDICATIONS:

Some surgeons recommend operations for all kidney stones. Most surgeons, however, think that operations to remove kidney stones are indicated only if they are causing kidney failure, or if they will not pass through the ureter and into the bladder in a reasonable period of time. But how long should one wait for a stone to pass? Large stones are less likely to pass, so operations may be indicated earlier for them. For most small stones, however, waiting a few days is reasonable, especially if the stone is progressing down the tube.

BENEFITS:

Relief of pain and discomfort and prevention of damage to the kidneys.

COMPLICATIONS:

1. Unnecessary operations because of eagerness to operate for stones that might otherwise pass without surgery.
2. All the complications of surgery and anesthesia discussed in Chapters Two and Six.
3. Damage to the ureter during surgery could obstruct urine flow resulting in kidney damage.

ALTERNATIVES:

The first alternative to operations for kidney stones is simply to wait for the stone to pass. One must avoid rushing into unnecessary operations when a kidney stone might pass harmlessly.

YOUR DECISION:

Knowing that most stones will pass, you can ask questions about your own particular case, and if it seems reasonable, you can postpone operation, allowing ample time for the stone to pass before agreeing to an operation.

Prostate Gland Operations

The male prostate gland encircles the urethra, the tube leading from the urinary bladder to the exterior of the body. Enlargement of the prostate gland obstructs the urethra, first causing increased frequency of urination, loss of the force of urinary stream, dribbling, intermittency, and finally complete obstruction of the flow of urine from the bladder.

Prostate trouble can result from benign enlargement or from cancer. By rectal examination, doctors can actually feel the prostate gland and can estimate on the basis of firmness and shape whether the gland is benign or malignant. A biopsy can provide additional information about the nature of swelling of the prostate gland.

When the gland enlarges to cause significant obstruction of the urethra, or when evidence of cancer is found, removal of the prostate gland is recommended. This can be performed either with a special instrument (cystoscope), looking through the urethra into the bladder, or through an incision into the abdomen.

INDICATIONS:

1.   Obstruction of the urethra.
2.   Cancer of the prostate gland.

BENEFITS:

1.   Restoration of normal urine flow.
2.   Cure of cancer.

COMPLICATIONS:

1.   All the complications of surgery and anesthesia described in Chapters Two and Six.
2.   Uncontrollable hemorrhage.
3.   Impotency, occurring especially with complete prostate removal through the abdomen.

ALTERNATIVES:

1.   If benign prostate disease is not completely obstructing the urethra, some patients can control their urination by avoiding excessive fluid intake and urinating frequently to prevent the bladder from becoming distended.
2.   Hormone therapy is also valuable for treating cancer of the prostate.

YOUR DECISION:

Operations to remove the prostate gland are variable and depend upon individual patients. You should ask about the particulars of your own case. You should remember, however, that there is no need to rush into an operation if your prostate is benign, your kidneys are functioning normally, and you can control urination with reasonable comfort. In all cases, the nature and the extent of operation, including side effects, should be discussed thoroughly with your doctor before you agree to prostate operation.

Thyroid Surgery

One of the most famous surgeons in the United States has said that the thyroid gland should never be removed, even for cancer. He shows convincingly that careful diagnosis coupled with medical therapy not only gives excellent results for thyroid diseases but also avoids all the complications of surgery. Many surgeons do not agree, however, and they continue to perform surgery upon the thyroid gland, especially for cancer.

Thyroid gland surgery is usually performed to treat swellings or tumors of the gland. Certain lumps can form on the thyroid gland either because of iodine deficiency or because of tumors. Most surgeons still operate on the thyroid gland if nodules are suspected of being malignant. Radioactive scanning can help to determine malignancy of thyroid nodules. If a nodule is radioactively "hot," it is considered more benign, if it is "cold," it is considered possibly malignant. Still, there is uncertainty, and often biopsy operations are performed to remove that portion of thyroid containing nodules. The tissue is then examined under the microscope to decide about malignancy. If malignancy is found, more extensive operations are designed to cure the cancer.

Surgeons who disagree with that traditional approach to thyroid nodules point out that thyroid cancer itself is most often a relatively benign disease, and that medications can produce results as good as surgery. So, they argue, instead of major operations to determine the nature of nodules, simple needle biopsies to remove tiny portions of tissue for examination will suffice. Then appropriate medications can be given.

INDICATIONS:

Obviously the indications for thyroid surgery vary widely. Recent reports about medical treatment for thyroid disease, including cancer, raise questions about whether any surgery except needle biopsy is ever indicated for the thyroid gland. Traditionally, thyroid surgery has been indicated for excisional biopsy followed by radical surgery if cancer is found, and for severe, uncontrollable cases of hyperthyroidism.

BENEFITS:

Surgery of the thyroid gland can offer definite diagnoses of nodules, cures for cancer, removal of swelling of the neck, and relief of the symptoms of hyperthyroidism.

COMPLICATIONS:

1. All the complications of surgery and anesthesia described in Chapters Two and Six.
2. Severance of the nerves to the vocal cords, resulting in hoarseness, voice weakness, or even severe breathing difficulties.

ALTERNATIVES:

Medications are available to control hormonal disturbances associated with benign thyroid disease. Medical treatment is also effective to treat benign and malignant tumors of the thyroid gland.

YOUR DECISION:

Just knowing that alternatives are available, you may decide to accept medical management of your thyroid condition rather than risking complications of major surgery. You may have to be persistent, perhaps even traveling to a medical center where such treatment is offered. On the other hand, you may prefer to have an operation, reasoning that since the vast majority of surgeons still advocate surgery for the thyroid gland, that decision is on the safer side.

Tonsillectomy (Adenoidectomy and Ear Canal Tubes)

As mentioned in Chapter Five, tonsillectomy is probably the operation most frequently performed unnecessarily. That is partly because the indications for tonsillectomy are so vague. Recently a "blue ribbon" panel was convened by the National Institute of Health to establish national standards for tonsillectomy. After weeks of argument, the panel was disbanded because the "experts" could not even agree about the actual purpose of tonsillectomy in the first place. The American public will have to wait another indeterminate period of time to find out whether or not their children require tonsillectomy.

The operation involves removing some of the soft, pink almond-shaped tissue on either side of the throat. Usually the adenoids, similar tissue behind the palate, are also removed. Additionally, now doctors are inserting little plastic tubes through patients' eardrums to try to prevent further infections of the inner ear.

INDICATIONS:

1. Indications for tonsillectomy, adenoidectomy, and ear canal tubes are not clearly defined.

2. Some doctors believe that tonsillectomy is good treatment for frequent sore throats in children, even without any complications of ear or sinus problems.

3. The most conservative doctors think tonsillectomy should be performed only if the tonsils are so bad they are actually blocking the airway or if rare malignant tumors are present. If these conservative indications were followed, the frequency of tonsillectomy would drop to 1 percent of what it is today.

BENEFITS:

The benefits of tonsillectomy are disputed. Proponents say that the operation reduces the incidence of throat infections, inner ear infections, loss of hearing, and mastoiditis, all of which can impair children's maturation and schoolwork. Opponents argue that less than 10 percent of children benefit from the operation and point out the risks involved. They add that tonsillitis is a self-limiting disease since almost all children grow out of the problem by the age of eight or ten years.

COMPLICATIONS:

1. Unnecessary operations because of eagerness to treat disease surgically when more conservative measures could give desirable effects.

2. Probably at least 20 percent of children who undergo tonsillectomy have complications of some kind.

3. Failure to obtain desired results—some children continue to have sore throats and ear problems despite tonsillectomy.

4. Hemorrhage—one of the most frequent and dreaded complications of tonsillectomy. A day or two after operation, blood begins to pour from the child's mouth. Aspiration of blood into the lungs is not rare under these circumstances. Cauterization and rehospitalization is usually necessary.

5. Drug and anesthetic reactions.

6. The psychological reactions to tonsillectomy deserve the most careful consideration. They are not as obvious as physical problems, but they can be even more destructive. The effects of frightening hospitalization and painful operations on the personalities of children are immeasurable. Some psychiatrists have estimated that 21 percent of children undergoing tonsillectomy suffer significant harmful effects upon later emotional development.

ALTERNATIVES:

1. Not having the operation at all, waiting for natural maturation and for children to grow out of the problem.

2.   Getting a second opinion before agreeing to surgery, especially from a pediatrician who is less likely to encourage surgery.

3.   More vigorous medical management, and especially preventive measures.

YOUR DECISION:

Think it over and use some common sense. After all, since you know that most children grow out of the disease, you might resolve to treat your children's infections more carefully, especially getting early treatment and trying to prevent exposure to upper respiratory infections. If the doctors disagree so vehemently, some saying that tonsillectomy should be reduced 99 percent, you will certainly need to exercise your own good judgment about whether to subject your child to tonsillectomy.

Trauma Surgery

Treatment of injuries to the human body may be the pinnacle of surgical accomplishment. In no other area of illness has surgery so much to offer. Serious damage to nerves, arteries, tendons, joints, and all internal organs can be repaired by prompt and appropriate surgical intervention. Some surgeons have specialized in injuries, and trauma centers have been established in most major metropolitan areas.

INDICATIONS:

Injury of any structure of the body either by blunt trauma, such as automobile accidents, or by penetrating wounds inflicted by knives or bullets. Skill and judgment are required to determine whether wounds might be just bruises or simple fractures or whether disruption of internal organs has occurred.

BENEFITS:

Repair of injuries can reverse events that might otherwise

have caused death or lifelong disabilities.

COMPLICATIONS:

1.   All the complications of surgery and anesthesia discussed in Chapters Two and Six.

2.   Mismanagement of injuries either by waiting too long to proceed with definitive repair or by rushing into operations for lesions that do not require surgery.

3.   Mismanagement of injuries in facilities in which qualified surgeons are not promptly available to provide emergency treatment for all problems found in victims of trauma.

ALTERNATIVES:

After severe injuries there are few alternatives to surgical care. Qualified surgeons must decide whether operations are necessary.

YOUR DECISION:

As you can imagine, lying on a stretcher in an emergency room following a serious injury, you may not be in any condition to make involved judgmental decisions. However, you should try to use some common sense. Obviously, if you are in shock and seriously injured, you will have little choice except to follow the judgment of the doctors. However, if your blood pressure is all right, if you feel pretty good, and the doctors are indefinite, you may want to choose to be transferred to your own hospital or to a trauma center. Better still, you might think about these problems ahead of time, ask about hospitals and doctors in your community, and have a plan in mind about where and how you might wish to be treated in case of serious injury.

Tubal Ligation

Tubal ligation refers to the method of female sterilization in which the Fallopian tubes, the conduits that lead from the ovaries to the womb (uterus), are cut and tied so that eggs can no longer pass through to be fertilized by sperm. These operations can be accomplished during other operations, such as cesarean section. When they are performed as separate procedures for sterilization, tubal ligations can be performed either through an incision on the abdominal wall, or by peritoneoscopy (see Endoscopy), using an instrument inserted through a small opening on the abdomen, through which the organs can be visualized and the Fallopian tubes cut and tied.

INDICATIONS:

Female sterilization.

BENEFITS:

Reliable birth control.

COMPLICATIONS:

1.   All the complications of surgery and anesthesia discussed in Chapters Two and Six.
2.   Injury to other organs and uncontrollable hemorrhage are immediate technical errors and require urgent major operations to repair the damage.
3.   Failure to achieve desired results—if the tubes are not adequately tied, sterilization is not accomplished.

ALTERNATIVES:

Other methods of birth control.

YOUR DECISION:

Recognizing the possible complications of tubal ligations, and the alternative methods of birth control, you should come to a careful decision about whether you wish to undergo tubal ligation.

Ulcer Operations, Duodenal

The causes of peptic ulcer disease are unknown. Emotions play a major role, but physical factors such as stomach acidity are also important. Most operations for ulcers of the duodenum become necessary because patients do not follow medical regimens carefully or diligently enough to heal their ulcers. Furthermore, except for brief counseling, measures to treat the emotional component of ulcer disease are all too often neglected by doctors. For some patients the usual antacid regimens are enough. For others psychotherapy and a change in lifestyle would help greatly. However, exercise, yoga, meditation, and other holistic health measures to heal ulcer disease have not been adequately studied or practiced. If ulcer disease could be controlled by complete health programs for emotional and physical health, most operations for peptic ulcers would be unnecessary.

Various operations have been developed for ulcers, but they all have one primary aim—to lower the acid in the stomach. Cure rates are higher with some of the complicated operations, but so are the complications and mortality rates. The simplest operations—just cutting the nerves to the stomach and opening up the channel into the duodenum—have very low complication and mortality rates, but the recurrence rate of ulcers is high. Obviously, patients who are advised to have operations for ulcers should discuss all these variables with their doctors.

Rarely, peptic ulcers can be caused by certain hormone disorders. Operations in those cases are to correct the offending endocrine glands.

INDICATIONS:

1.   Failure of medical management is the most common reason for operating for ulcer disease. All too often, however, the medical management itself has not been adequate. Some patients neglect their own health. Others are never offered adequate instruction for complete programs, including physical and emotional components of their illness.

2.   Hemorrhage from ulcers can be severe, necessitating urgent operations. Usually, however, hemorrhage stops in a short

period of time and there is time for reassessment. After hemorrhage, some patients may begin to realize the importance of their health program and start afresh with a more vigorous regimen to prevent recurrence of hemorrhage and to heal their ulcers.

3.   Perforation of an ulcer through the wall of the duodenum, spilling intestinal juices into the peritoneal cavity, usually requires an urgent operation. However, some doctors have successfully treated perforations with stomach suction, intravenous fluids, and antibiotics. If operation for perforation is performed, the extent of the surgery varies. Some surgeons advocate simple closure of the perforation, pointing out that most patients will never require further surgery. Other surgeons perform more extensive, definitive operations at the time of the first operation.

4.   Surgery may become necessary for other problems associated with ulcers, such as obstruction of the intestine or involvement of adjacent organs.

BENEFITS:

1.   Relief of indigestion and pain associated with peptic ulcer disease.

2.   Lifesaving treatment for complications of ulcers, such as hemorrhage or perforation.

3.   In rare cases, resolution of underlying endocrine disorders can result from the surgical management of peptic ulcer disease.

COMPLICATIONS:

1.   All the complications of surgery and anesthesia discussed in Chapters Two and Six.

2.   Severe indigestion, pain, vomiting, diarrhea, and malnutrition can occur following operations for ulcer disease.

ALTERNATIVES:

In cases of emergency because of hemorrhage or perforation there is little opportunity to choose alternatives, except to take the chance that the hemorrhage will stop or the perforation will heal with proper medical care. In most cases, there is ample time for careful evaluation of all the variables and for patients to decide whether to have operations. For some, a more vigorous program of medical and emotional management will improve ulcer disease.

YOUR DECISION:

Most operations for peptic ulcer disease come about because patients have not taken care of themselves adequately, either because they neglect their own health or because they have never been thoroughly advised about a complete program. If an operation is recommended for you, perhaps you should resolve to take better care of yourself. By starting a careful dedicated program of medical management, and perhaps investigating those areas not recommended by doctors—exercise, nutritional, and emotional programs—you might be able to avoid having an operation for peptic ulcer disease.

Ulcer Operations, Stomach

Ulcers of the stomach are different from ordinary duodenal peptic ulcers and demand a different approach. Whereas duodenal ulcers are benign, stomach ulcers can sometimes be malignant. Differences of opinions exist among doctors as to how to manage stomach ulcers, surgeons usually advocating a more aggressive operative approach because of the possibility of cancer, and internists encouraging medical management first so as to avoid unnecessary operations in patients with benign ulcers. Furthermore, once operation is deemed necessary, surgeons disagree about how extensive operations should be, some performing limited resections for cancer and others preferring more radical procedures, removing most of the stomach and adjacent organs. Statistics about different cure rates and mortality rates for the various operations are inconclusive.

INDICATIONS:

1. Hemorrhage or perforation of stomach ulcers.
2. Stomach ulcers that have been shown to be malignant.
3. Stomach ulcers that fail to heal with adequate medical management.

BENEFITS:

1. Relief of indigestion and pain caused by stomach ulcers.
2. Prevention of further complications of stomach ulcers.
3. Possible cure of stomach cancer.

COMPLICATIONS:

1. All the complications of surgery and anesthesia discussed in Chapters Two and Six.
2. Severe indigestion, pain, vomiting, diarrhea, weight loss, and malnutrition.

ALTERNATIVES:

1. For benign stomach ulcers, more careful medical management may heal the disease.
2. For stomach ulcers which are definitely or probably malignant, there are few alternatives to surgery. However, the extensiveness of the operations can vary.

YOUR DECISION:

You will need all the specific information about your illness before you can decide whether to have an operation for stomach ulcers. If the ulcer is most likely benign, however, you can choose to try vigorous medical management before agreeing to an operation.

Once you decide to have an operation, you should ask questions about how extensive your operation will be. Find out the statistics about the various operations and decide whether you want a radical or more simple procedure.

Varicose Vein Operations

Varicose veins, those wormlike protrusions on the legs, are usually the result of poor circulation because of inadequate valves in the veins of the legs up to the groin. Removing varicose veins to improve appearance is purely elective (see Cosmetic Surgery). Sometimes, however, poor circulation caused by these veins can result in inflammation (phlebitis), ankle swelling, ulceration of the skin, and chronic leg pain. Additionally, poor circulation in varicose veins can actually lead to decreased blood flow through the deeper veins of the legs, which itself can lead to deep vein phlebitis and blood clots. Removing varicose veins can actually improve circulation in the legs, thereby improving symptoms and preventing progression of skin or deep vein problems.

INDICATIONS:

    1.   Cosmetic improvement.
    2.   Significant impairment of circulation in the legs, resulting in skin ulcerations, ankle swelling, or pain.
    3.   Phlebitis.

BENEFITS:

    1.   Improvement in appearance.
    2.   Improvement in function allowing for more standing and walking.
    3.   Prevention of deep vein phlebitis and clots.

COMPLICATIONS:

    1.   All the complications of surgery and anesthesia discussed in Chapters Two and Six.
    2.   Recurrence—varicose veins can recur over a period of years if measures are not taken to continue to improve circulation in the legs.
    3.   Technical errors during operations have resulted in dam-

age to arteries or nerves. The operation is considered minor by many people, but skilled surgeons are required.

4.   If the deep leg veins are not adequate, the removal of the varicose veins could interrupt circulation, making symptoms worse instead of better. Care must be taken to insure that the deep veins of the legs are competent before varicose veins are removed.

ALTERNATIVES:

Improvement in venous circulation of the legs can be achieved in other ways. Just refraining from prolonged standing and elevating the legs intermittently can help a great deal. Elevating the legs and doing toe exercises for five or ten minutes three or four times a day can result in greatly improved circulation in the legs and reduction in varicose veins. Furthermore, elastic stockings fitted to the legs can effectively empty the varicose veins and divert the circulation to the deep veins, thereby accomplishing all the goals of operations.

YOUR CHOICE:

Knowing the alternatives are available, you might want to judge whether you have given nonoperative techniques a chance. You just might find that a careful program to improve your leg vein circulation will work and you can avoid the risks of an operation.

Vasectomy

Vasectomy, cutting and tying the sperm tubes, which lead from the testicles into the seminal vesicles inside the pelvis, has become a popular method of birth control. The operation is described as the simplest and safest reliable method of birth control known. Although the operation itself is relatively simple, there are some important ramifications. First of all, the procedure must be considered irreversible, because for those patients who change their minds later, less than 10 percent of attempts to reconstruct the tubes are successful. Additionally, some researchers have reported increased estrogen levels, loss of body muscle, and certain vague autoimmune responses in which patients form antibodies against their own body tissues. These findings suggest that there may be unknowns about the long-term affects of vasectomy.

INDICATIONS:

Voluntary male sterilization.

BENEFITS:

Reliable birth control.

COMPLICATIONS:

1. Swelling, hemorrhage, or infection in the scrotum.
2. Failure to achieve the desired results. Sometimes because of technical problems all the tubes from the testicles are not adequately tied and sperm can still travel through. In other rare cases, new channels form over a period of years, renewing male fertility.
3. Changes in hormone balance and autoimmune responses still not clearly understood. The long-term effects of these phenomena are unknown.
4. Psychological reactions, including guilt and impotency. These may be especially apparent in individuals with personal or religious doubts about the efficacy of vasectomy.

ALTERNATIVES:

Other methods of birth control.

YOUR DECISION:

Birth control is a matter of personal preference depending

upon desires, necessities, and beliefs. All the ramifications should be evaluated before seeking vasectomy.

Weight-reduction Operations

Obesity may be the number one health problem in the United States. Various methods of dieting become popular from time to time, and some doctors have even specialized in weight-reduction clinics. The overall efforts to reduce weight have been ineffective, however, and probably less than 1 percent of patients lose significant amounts of weight permanently. As in other areas of medical failures, surgeons sooner or later try to offer solutions. Operations for weight reduction actually short-circuit the intestine, so that instead of twenty-two feet of intestine to absorb food, only about one foot is available. After these operations, patients can continue to eat, but the ingested food is rushed through the shortened intestine and out of the body in the form of frequent, soft stools. Other weight reduction operations involve markedly reducing the size of the stomach, thereby decreasing the appetite. With these techniques, patients can lose weight at a rapid rate for a period of two or three years. After that, the intestine enlarges and becomes more efficient so that weight remains stable.

Weight-reduction operations inflict a profound physiological insult on the body, altering hormone balance, upsetting fluid and mineral balances, impairing kidney and liver function, and sometimes causing deep psychological disturbances. Patients should have complete physical and psychiatric evaluations before these operations.

INDICATIONS:

Severe, morbid obesity that cannot be controlled by dieting.

BENEFITS:

1. Weight loss.

2.   Improvement in other ailments, such as high blood pressure and diabetes.

COMPLICATIONS:

1.   All the complications of surgery and anesthesia discussed in Chapters Two and Six.
2.   Because candidates for these operations are already obese, the complication and death rates for these operations are higher than for most surgery.
3.   Other organ complications, such as the formation of gallstones.
4.   Some unusual complications, such as temporary loss of hair.
5.   Irreversible liver disease of unknown cause. A repeat operation to return the intestine to normal is required to save these patients' lives.
6.   A high incidence of wound infections and healing problems because of obesity.
7.   Failure to achieve the desired results—for unknown reasons some patients fail to lose significant amounts of weight.
8.   Severe mineral and hormonal imbalances.
9.   Psychological disturbances.

ALTERNATIVES:

Other methods of weight control.

YOUR DECISION:

These are dangerous operations with higher than usual death and complication rates. Many of the long-term effects are unknown. Patients should thoroughly evaluate the risks before deciding about these operations for weight control.

Index

About the Author

Dr. Myron K. Denney has been practicing medicine and surgery for eighteen years, and is a Fellow of the American College of Surgeons, the Association for Academic Surgeons, and the American College of Emergency Physicians. After his internship in 1960, he spent two years in Europe and the Near East working for NATO, and then traveled around the world visiting and working in missionary hospitals. In 1964, he was granted the Frederick Coller Award by the American College of Surgeons. He has published many medical articles and research papers in the *Journal of the American Medical Association* and other prestigious journals. His writing interests have also included such diverse subjects as liver and lung disease, worldwide cholera epidemics, scuba diving and off-road racing. Dr. Denney has served as an assistant professor of surgery on the medical staffs of three major universities. He is currently practicing and writing in New York City.

"An informative, readable guide to the mysteries of surgery. Readers should welcome Denney's outspoken comments. Because surgeons are traditionally an uncommunicative group, this book is an especially welcome aid to delineating patients' rights and expanding their knowledge."

—*Publishers Weekly*

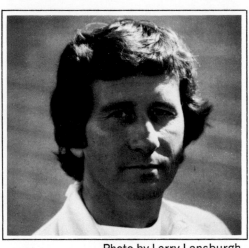

Photo by Larry Lansburgh

Dr. Myron K. Denney has been practicing medicine and surgery for eighteen years, and is a Fellow of the American College of Surgeons, the Association for Academic Surgeons, and the American College of Emergency Physicians. He has published many medical articles and scholarly papers in the *Journal of the American Medical Association, Archives of Surgery,* and other prestigious journals. He has served on the medical staff of three major universities and has been an emergency surgeon with the Children's Hospital of San Francisco and Vesper Memorial Hospital in San Leandro. Dr. Denney currently practices in New York City.

today press ®

GROSSET & DUNLAP
A FILMWAYS COMPANY
Publishers • New York

0-448-16549-X